PSYCHIATRY
MADE EASY®

PSYCHIATRY
MADE EASY®

T Anbu RNMSc (N) DEDN
Principal
Sri Vishnu College of Nursing
Bengaluru, Karnataka, India

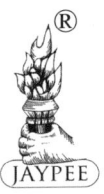

JAYPEE BROTHERS MEDICAL PUBLISHERS (P) LTD
New Delhi • London • Philadelphia • Panama

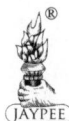 **Jaypee Brothers Medical Publishers (P) Ltd**

Headquarters
Jaypee Brothers Medical Publishers (P) Ltd
4838/24, Ansari Road, Daryaganj
New Delhi 110 002, India
Phone: +91-11-43574357
Fax: +91-11-43574314
Email: jaypee@jaypeebrothers.com

Overseas Offices

J.P. Medical Ltd
83 Victoria Street, London
SW1H 0HW (UK)
Phone: +44-2031708910
Fax: +02-03-0086180
Email: info@jpmedpub.com

Jaypee-Highlights Medical Publishers Inc
City of Knowledge, Bld. 237, Clayton
Panama City, Panama
Phone: +507-301-0496
Fax: +507-301-0499
Email: cservice@jphmedical.com

Jaypee Medical Inc
The Bourse
111 South Independence Mall East
Suite 835, Philadelphia, PA 19106, USA
Phone: + 267-519-9789
Email: joe.rusko@jaypeebrothers.com

Jaypee Brothers Medical Publishers (P) Ltd
17/1-B Babar Road, Block-B, Shaymali
Mohammadpur, Dhaka-1207
Bangladesh
Mobile: +08801912003485
Email: jaypeedhaka@gmail.com

Jaypee Brothers Medical Publishers (P) Ltd
Shorakhute, Kathmandu, Nepal
Phone: +00977-9841528578
Email: jaypee.nepal@gmail.com

Website: www.jaypeebrothers.com
Website: www.jaypeedigital.com

© 2014, Jaypee Brothers Medical Publishers

All rights reserved. No part of this book may be reproduced in any form or by any means without the prior permission of the publisher.

Inquiries for bulk sales may be solicited at: jaypee@jaypeebrothers.com

This book has been published in good faith that the contents provided by the author contained herein are original, and is intended for educational purposes only. While every effort is made to ensure accuracy of information, the publisher and the author specifically disclaim any damage, liability, or loss incurred, directly or indirectly, from the use or application of any of the contents of this work. If not specifically stated, all figures and tables are courtesy of the author. Where appropriate, the readers should consult with a specialist or contact the manufacturer of the drug or device.

Psychiatry Made Easy®

First Edition: **2014**

ISBN: 978-93-5090-967-6

Printed at Rajkamal Electric Press, Plot No. 2, Phase-IV, Kundli, Haryana.

Preface

"Money cannot make mental health."

There is no health without mental health. Mental disorders are major contribution to illness and premature death and are responsible for 13 percent of the global disease burden. With the global economic downturn, the risk of mental ill health is rising around the globe.

I hope this book *Psychiatry Made Easy* will help the students to understand the basic concepts in mental health and also they can use this knowledge in prevention of psychiatric disorders and to maintain mental health.

This book is arranged in a rather simplified language with detailed tables so as to make it much easier and simpler and thus create an interest in the students for this subject.

In this book, each chapter has been dealt with proper care with regard to relevancy and narrated by systematic sequence.

I am sure that this book will serve as perfect teaching guide for the teacher and good reference book for the students. It is also useful for paramedical and social workers who are providing care for mentally ill persons in various settings.

T Anbu

Acknowledgments

As someone has rightly stated, 'Dream a thousand dreams and actualize at least a few'. This work is the realization of a long-cherished dream. Every creative inspiration comes from the creator and even the minute creative action is a participation in the creative work of Almightly. The little knowledge which has been imparted to me during my studies, and the greater information and experiences. I received during my teaching profession, inspired and enabled me to complete this book.

I wish to acknowledge the help I have received from many sources without which this work would not have been completed.

I am greatly indebted to Mr S Jagadeesh, Chairman, Sri Vishnu College of Nursing, Bengaluru, for his goodwill and encouragement. I am extremely thankful to my friends Mr G Loganathan, Vice-Principal, Sri Venkateshwara College of Nursing, Bengaluru and Mr Gopinath, MSc (N), Ireland, for their constant motivation.

I would like to acknowledge and thank all my family members especially my wife Mrs Kavitha, who gave continuous cooperation and valuable assistance in bringing out this book.

Last but not least, I would also like to thank Shri Jitendar P Vij (Group Chairman), Mr Ankit Vij (Managing Director), Mr Tarun Duneja (Director-Publishing) and other staff of M/s Jaypee Brothers Medical Publishers (P) Ltd, New Delhi, India, and Mr Santhosh Kumar, Author Coordinator, for their constant support and cooperation during preparation of manuscript and finally undertaking this publication.

Contents

1. **Introduction**   1
   History of psychiatry *1*
   History of psychiatric nursing *6*
   Prevalence of mental disorders *7*
   Definition *9*
   Criteria for good mental health *9*
   Causes of mental disorders *9*
   Classification of mental disorders *10*
   Principles of mental health nursing *12*
   The interdisciplinary treatment team *13*
   Preventive psychiatry *15*
   Community facilities available in India *16*

2. **Conceptual Models**   17
   Personality *17*
   Freud theory *18*
   Psychosexual stage theory *20*
   Erik Erikson's 8 stages of psychosocial development *21*
   Kohlberg's theory of moral development *23*
   Peplau's interpersonal theory *23*
   Piaget's theory of cognitive development *24*

3. **Mental Health Assessment**   26
   History collection *26*
   Mental status examination (MSE) *28*
   Mini mental state examination (MMSE) *31*
   Neurological examination *32*
   Psychological tests *38*

4. **Therapeutic Relationship**   39
   Communication *39*
   Interpersonal communication *40*
   Johari window *46*
   Therapeutic impasses *48*

5. **Psychotic Disorders**   52
   Functional psychosis or schizophrenia *52*
   Mood disorders *59*
   Other types of mood disorders *60*
   Treatment of bipolar disorder *62*
   Organic mental disorders *67*
   Other psychotic disorders *71*

6. Neurotic Disorders — 76
Anxiety 76
Phobic disorder 78
Obsessive compulsive disorder 81
Hysterical neurosis (dissociative and conversion disorder) 84
Post-traumatic stress disorder 86
The somatoform disorders 86
Premenstrual syndrome (PMS) 87
Hyperventilation syndrome 89
Irritable bowel syndrome (IBS) 90

7. Psychoactive Substance Use Disorder — 93
Psychoactive drugs 93
Alcohol use disorder 96
Opioids and related disorder 101
Cocaine and related disorder 104
Cannabis and related disorders 106
Caffeine-related disorder 106
Amphetamines and related disorder 109
Inhalants use disorder 110
Hallucinogens and related disorder 111

8. Psychophysiological Disorder — 114
Anorexia nervosa 114
Bulimia nervosa 115
Other eating disorders 115
Somatization disorder 119
Sleep disorders 121

9. Personality Disorder — 129
Types of personality disorders 129

10. Psychosexual Disorder — 134
The sexual response cycle 134

11. Childhood Mental Disorder — 140
Mental retardation 142
Common types of behavior problems with mental retardation 144
Classification of mental retardation 145
Difference in mental retardation and mental illness 148
Autism spectrum disorders 148
Attention deficit hyperactivity disorder 150
Conduct disorder 156
Elimination disorder 157
Encopresis 158

12. Emergency Psychiatry — 162
Emergency 162
Suicide 162
Stupor 164
Excitement (violence) 165

Refusal of food 165
Rape 166
Other psychotic emergencies 166

13. **Legal Aspects of Psychiatry** — 167
    Indian Lunacy Act (16th March 1912) 167
    The Mental Health Act, 1987 167
    Rights of mentally ill clients 170
    Legal responsibilities of a mentally ill person 170
    The narcotic Drugs and Psychotropic
    *   Substances Act (NDPSA), 1985 171*

14. **Biopsychosocial Therapies** — 172
    Historical development of psychopharmocology 172
    Antipsychotic drugs 173
    Antimanic drugs 175
    Antidepressant drugs 176
    Anti-anxiety drugs 177
    Psychotherapy 178
    Behavior therapy techniques based on classical conditioning 180
    Cognitive behavior therapy (CBT) 185
    Milieu therapy 188
    Therapeutic community 191
    Family therapy 194
    Marital therapy (couples therapy) 195
    Occupational therapy (OT) 195
    Music therapy 196
    Dance/movement therapy 197
    Psychodrama 197
    Recreational therapy 198
    Light therapy 199
    Electroconvulsive therapy 199
    Alternative approaches to mental health treatment 202

15. **Community Mental Health** — 205
    National mental health program 205
    Psychiatric rehabilitation 208
    Institutionalization vs deinstitutionalization 211

16. **Mental Disorders for Special People** — 212
    Mental disorders in women 212
    Mental disorders in elders 223

17. **Crisis Situation** — 230
    Stress and coping 230
    Grief 235
    Crisis 238

Appendices — 243

Glossary — 257

Index — 267

Chapter 1

Introduction

HISTORY OF PSYCHIATRY

Introduction

To understand psychiatry today, it is important to understand how the human knowledge and process of thinking evolved. The object of psychiatry involves not only the biological studies but also many of psychological, psychosocial and sociocultural nature. The historic evolution of psychiatric knowledge shows that psychiatry and medicine shared common origins and the objective and field of study of both sciences were always in the terrain of clinical manifestations.

Ancient History

Prior to the age of Greek culture, physical and psychological assumptions of the primitive man were based in magical and intuitive assumptions, and were the activity of priests and sorceres. Nevertheless, in ancient Egypt there were surgeons that operated the brain and in ancient China, 30 centuries ago, there were some knowledge about pharmacology and pharmacotherapy.

The Greco-Roman Culture

Hippocrates (460–377 BC) believed that epilepsy (known as "Sacred Disease") was a condition with natural origins in the brain. He also believed that the human body was filled with four basic substances, called humors, which are in balance when a person is healthy. To Hippocrates, diseases resulted from a imbalance of these humors (Humorism). He also defined three types of mental diseases: *Phrenitis* (mental disorder with fever), *Mania* (mental disorder with agitation, without fever) and *Melancholia* (chronic mental disorder, without agitation or fever).

Asclepiades of Bithynia (124 or 129–40 BC) was a greek physician who worked with mental medicine. He founded his medical practice on a modification of the atomic theory (Atomism), according to which disease and psychological phenomena result from irregular or inharmonious motion of the corpuscles of the body. He believed that the soul had no specific localization (resulting from the concentration of perceptive functions) and that mental diseases were a consequence of disturbances of the passions.

Galen (AD 129–ca. 200 or 216) at the dawn of the Christian era stated that the nervous system was the center of sensation, motility and mental functions and that psychiatric disorders had cerebral origins. Galen was the first to state that *"hysteria"* should not be considered exclusive of the female gender.

Erasistratus of Chios (304 BC–250 BC), known as the father of physiology and Herophilus (335–280 BC), known as the father of anatomy studied the sensitive and motor nerves with important considerations on the Ventricular system. Aulus Cornelius Celsus (ca 25 BC–ca 50) was the first to designate the psychiatric diseases by *"Insania"*.

Psychiatry and Greek Philosophy

Aristotle (384 BC–322 BC) can be considered the true father of psychology. He studied sensations and inteligence, wrote considerations on the imagination, judgment, logic and memory and stated that the psychological operations were functions of material organs. Aristotle defended the "methodology of reason" and founded the *"Peripatetic School"* that can be considered the founding of psychotherapy and psychopedagogy.

Socrates (469 BC–399 BC) was the first to defend the supremacy of the faculty of "thinking", which he considered the best way to achieve the *"knowledge of yourself"* (*Nosce te ipsum*). During the socratic period, philosophy became a true anthropology.

Plato (428/427 BC–348/347 BC), defined the world of "ideas", a monist concept (body and nature are manifestations of the ideal essence) that dominated the western philosophy. With Plato and Aristotle philosophy reached the "systematic" period, with the elaboration of concepts (Theory of Forms), to which one can relate the laws of association (Aristotelian logic) and the definition of the scientific body that years later became science and psychology. The Greek culture and philosophy were the main source of knowledge over the nature of the psychological phenomena. It is because of this impact that many designations and terminologies universally used in psychiatry have greek routes: *schizophrenia, paranoia, oligophrenia*, among others. This is also the reason why Psychoanalysis used many concepts of the hellenic civilization, such as *Oedipus complex*.

Christianity and Psychiatry

As the christianism spread, beliefs that mental illnesses were manifestations of divine rage became common.

Augustine of Hippo (354–430), studied memory and consciousness, but his religiosity would not allow that his observations could go against the supernatural concept of the psychiatric disease. He believed that men had, since birth, an original inclination to sin that was transmitted through the concupiscence (lust) that accompanied sexual reproduction, weakening the will and making humanity a *massa damnata* (condemned crowd). This observation later influenced psychoanalysis and phenomenology.

During the Middle Ages, psychiatric disorders were once again in the land of the supernatural and the most common therapeutic procedures were exorcisms and casting outs, to free the body of evil spirits. Examples of the beliefs at time can be found at the *"Malleus Maleficarum* (The Hammer of Witches)", written by two dominican priests (Heinrich Kraemer and James Sprenger) in 1484. The *Malleus Maleficarum* is a book that describes the Devil's influence on witches (through lust), how to identify witchcraft and how witches should be judged and punished. The book constitutes a manual of pornography and detailed psychopathology.

Despite the superstition that dominated those times, the first *"asylums"* or mental hospitals were opened in Europe, at the end of the first millenium. The first ones were the colony of Geel in Belgium (850) and the Bethlem Royal Hospital in London. Unfortunately, the concept degenerated progressevely and the mentally ill, the poor, and those abandoned by their families were send to *"Hospices"*, charitable institutions that were a mix between assistance and reclusion facilities. Criminals were also sent to the Hospices and all interns were under the same rules of repression and monitoring: foot-irons, whips and food deprivation.

Some philosophers, however, brought some advance to psychiatry during the Middle Ages. Thomas Aquinas (1225–7 March, 1274) influenced by Aristotle, studied psychology and created the *Thomism*, a type of neo-Aristotelism. During the Renaissance, Paracelsus (1493–1541) advocated that mental illness was a disorder of the internal substance of the body, which was intimately connected to the soul and that the body's ability to "heal itself" should be reinforced. Thus, Paracelsus can be considered the first psychotherapist.

Johann Weyer (1514–1588) was a Dutch physician and wrote the *De Praestigiis Daemonum et Incantationibus ac Venificiis*. He stated that mental illnesses were not supernatural conditions and that witches should be treated as psychiatric patients. Unfortunately, those advances were isolated and only at the end of the XVII Century, there was an increase in scientific interpretation of the "spiritual diseases".

Rationalism

Thomas Willis (1621–1675) was an anatomist and neurologist who described the Circle of Willis (a circle of arteries that supply blood to the brain), general paralysis (syphilis) and Myasthenia gravis. Willis also stated that some youngsters, during puberty presented with a condition of "stupidity", a clinical state that was later related to what came to be known as schizophrenia.

The French Revolution and Philippe Pinel

The humanistic ideas from the French Revolution, combating the degrading conception of mental disorders achieved their peak in the gesture of the French physician Philippe Pinel (1745–1826). Pinel's ideas were published in his *Treatise on Insanity (Traité médico-philosophique sur l'aliénation mentale; ou*

la manie), that can be considered as the first Antipsychiatry book. Pinel was the first who seriously tried to classify mental disorders, which he grouped into four categories: "manias" or general delusions, "melancholies" or "exclusive delusions", "dementia" and "idiots". His studies and reformations constituted the *First psychiatric revolution*, introducing concepts of morality and liberty.

His gesture had wide repercusions and influenced many in other countries, such as WIlliam Tuke, a tea merchant who created the first *retreat* or humanized asylum, in the proximity of York, England.

During the century of Iluminism, many contributions to modern psychiatry must be recognized, such as those of William Cullen (1712–1790), a psychiatrist from Edinburgh who whote one of the first classifications of mental disorders based in scientific evidence. The second half of the XVIII century was a decisive time in the maturation of the psychiatric scientific method and the most prominent figure was, undoubtebly, Immanuel Kant (1724–1804), creator of transcendental philosophy.

Romantism and Neurophysiology

At the French school, the study and treatment of neurosis was a terrain of great disput due to the works of the neurologist Jean-Martin Charcot (1825–1893), who studied hypnosis and hysteria. Charcot considered that these were due to an organic instability in the central nervous system (CNS). This concept was disputed by the Nancy school, that defended the "suggestionable nature" of those phenomena. On Charcot's side was Pierre Janet, a psychiatrist who created the term "Psycasthenia" for that organic debility. Janet hypnotised many patients and discovered that, under hypnoses, they could remember traumatic events and that those memories could help in the cure of mental disorders. This technique of "emotional discharge" was discovered and described almost at the same time by the school of Viena (Sigmund Freud).

Natural sciences also had great influence on the psychiatric method of that time, especially the works of Charles Darwin and Louis Pasteur. These and many other authors' works constituted the begining of the *Modern Era of Medicine*. Most psychiatrists during the second half of the XIX century began to look for an organic cause of mental disorders and tried to find objective histological relationships between them.

Kraepelin (1856–1926) studied the "hard" psychiatry (psychoses and asylums) while Freud (1856–1939) studied the "light" psychiatry (neurosis and psychiatric office). Kraepelin gave importance to data from clinical observation, rather than anatomo-pathological. With Freud, personal biography gains importance and the acquired psychological factors have a predominant role on the elaboration and valorisation of the disorder.

In Italy, the anthropologist Cesare Lombroso (1836–1909) created important concepts to Criminology, such as "psychological degeneration" and tried to define the "born criminal", the "criminally insane" and the "moral imbeciles". Lombroso rejected the established concept that crime was a characteristic trait of

human nature and used concepts of physiognomy, eugenics, psychiatry and social darwinism to create a theory of anthropological criminology.

Due to works of authors such as Charcot, Meinert, Wernicke, Alzheirmer and Pick, this period of the XIX century can be called the *Golden Age of Neuropsychiatry*.

Early XX Century and Psychotherapy

Adding to the impact on the scientific method that came from the naturalists and neuropsychiatrists, another came, this time, from the revolutionary sociological concepts of the *"historical materialism"* of Karl Marx and Friedrick Engels, that deeply changed the structure of social relations. Psychiatry was also influenced by positivism, which characterized the late XIX century and persisted until the First World War.

The discovery of the syphilis agent, the bacteria Treponema pallidum inclined psychiatry even more to an organicist orientation. However, with the spread of freudian theories, the conceptual bipolarity of psychiatry became more accentuated. In the between Wars, psychiatry was divided between two irreconcilable theories: the first of organic and the second of psychological nature, that considered disturbing emotional mechanisms and conflict situations as main causes of mental disorders.

In organic psychiatry, genetic studies started in Germany, at the *Institut für Erbforschun* or German Research Institute for Psychiatry in Munich. Studies developed there proved that several nosographic entities described by Kraepelin (specifically endogenous psychoses) had hereditary basis. Meanwhile, Ernst Kretschmer (1888–1964) wrote *Body Structure and Character*, in which certain physical properties in the face, skull and body were linked to personalities and mental disorders.

In psychoanalysis, some of the authors that contributed to the systematization and divulgence of psychoanalytical concepts were Adler, Jung, Melanie Klein and Sandor Ferenczi.

In 1911, Bleuler created the term "Schizophrenia" (morbid process of personality split) to replace the term *dementia praecox* or "precocious dementia" created by Bénédict Morel in the XIX century and used by Kraepelin

The works of Ivan Pavlov describing the conditioned reflex and reflexology increased the dispute of non-existing etiopathological specificity of psychiatric disorders. By then, the medical model was accepted but psychogenic factors and interpersonal relations were also defended as causes for psychological decompensation. At the base of this relationship were, once more, philosophical foundations. Willy Mayer-Gross was an enthusiast of phenomenology in psychiatry, however, it was the work of Karl Jaspers, published in 1913, the most significative in changing the psychiatric perspective. Jaspers established a synthesis between the philosophical process and the psychiatric knowledge, creating a systematic methodology to approach all mental disorders in two ways: The explicative method (*erklären*) and the comprehensive method (*versthehen*).

Kurt Schneider was another author of great repercussion, contributting to the nosographic systematization of psychiatric entities and to the understanding of schizophrenia.

As for treatment, the first attempt to extend the biophysical knowledge was made by Julius von Wagner Jauregg, who administered malaria medication to psychiatric manifestations of syphilis. With the isolation of insulin in 1922, the first experiments with insulin shock therapy in schizophrenic patients started in 1933 with Manfred Sakel. Also in 1933, the first therapeutic effects of convulsions in schizophrenia were described by Ladislay von Meduna. Egas Moniz, in 1935, developed the first psychosurgery intervention by performing the first lobothomy. Electroconvulsive therapy was used for treatment for the first time in 1938.

In 1952, Jean Delay and Pierre Deniker reported the effects of chlorpromazine in psychotic patients, thus began the psychopharmacological revolution for the treatment of psychiatric conditions. This period is referred to as the *Second Psychiatric Revolution*.

The *Third Psychiatric Revolution* began in the 60's in United States, from the cultural anthropology, consisting of a movement of preventive character (in mental health). This continues to be one of the main aspects of american psychiatric today.

Second Half 20th Century

These period experienced the reemergency of biological psychiatry. Psychopharmacology became part of psychiatry with the discovery of the first neurotransmitter by Otto Loewi: Acetylcholine.

Radiology and image diagnosis was first used as a psychiatric tool in 1980. The discovery of the efficacy of chlorpromazine in the treatment of Schizophrenia in 1952 revolutionized the theurapeutical approach of the condition, just as lithium carbonate revolutionized treatment of euphoria and depression in Bipolar Disorder, in 1948.

When psychosocial problems seemed to be the cause, psychotherapy seemed to be the "cure"; and once more genetics was thought to have a fundamental role in mental disease. In 1995, genes that contribute to schizophrenia were found in chromosome 6 and genes related to bipolar disorder in chromosomes 18 and 21.

HISTORY OF PSYCHIATRIC NURSING

- In the 1840s, Florence Nightingale made an attempt to meet the needs of psychiatric patients with proper hygiene, better food, light and ventilation and the use of drugs to chemically restrain violent and aggressive patients.
- Linda Richards, the first psychiatric nurse graduated in the United States in 1882 from Boston City College.
- In 1913, Johns Hopkins University was the first college of nursing in the United States to offer psychiatric nursing as part of its general curriculum.

Introduction

- The first psychiatric nursing textbook, *Nursing Mental Diseases* was authored by Harriet Bailey, in 1920.
- The registration of psychiatric nurses was done by 1920 in the UK and degree courses in psychiatric nursing began in the USA.
- Short training courses of three to six months were conducted in Ranchi in 1921, which were recognized by the Royal Medical Psychological Association.
- For the first time in India, 11 British nurses along with one matron were brought from the UK to work in the mental hospital at Ranchi in the 1930s.
- During 1948–50 four nurses were sent to the UK by Government of India for mental health nursing diploma.
- From 1943, the Chennai Government organized a three months' psychiatric nursing course (subsequently stopped in 1964), for male nursing students at the Mental Hospital, Chennai (in lieu of midwifery).
- During 1954, Manzil Medical Health center, Lucknow gave psychiatric nursing orientation course of 4–6 weeks duration.
- Government of India decided to start training psychiatric nurses during 1953–54 and started the first organized course at All India Institute of Mental Health (presently NIMHANS).
- Psychiatric nursing was included in the basic nursing curriculum by the International Council of Nurses in 1961.
- In 1963, President John F Kennedy in United States passed the Community Mental Health Act which proposed the deinstitutionalization of mentally ill persons.
- In fourth century AD, during the period of Emperor Ashoka, hospitals with 15 beds for mentally ill with two male and two female nurses. In 1964–65, Psychiatric nursing was included in curriculum.
- In 1964–1965, the Indian Nursing Council (INC) made it a requirement to integrate psychiatric nursing in the nursing diploma and degree courses.
- In 1967, a separate Psychiatric Nursing Committee was formed in the Trained Nurses Association of India.
- Diploma in Psychiatric Nursing is conducted in three institutions in India.
- Master of Psychiatric Nursing (MPN) program is conducted in many institutions.
- Doctoral program in psychiatric nursing (PhD) at NIMHANS, Bangalore.

PREVALENCE OF MENTAL DISORDERS

National-level data on the prevalence of mental disorders are not available. However, a meta-analysis of 13 epidemiological studies yielded an estimated prevalence rate of 5.8%. Organic psychosis (0.04%), alcohol/drug dependence (0.69%), schizophrenia (0.27%), affective disorders (1.23%), neurotic disorders (2.07%), mental retardation (0.69%) and epilepsy (0.44%) were common diagnoses.

12 Morbidity was associated with residence (urban), gender (females), age group (35–44 years), marital status (married/widowed/divorced), socioeconomic status (lower) and family type (nuclear).

The Indian Government estimates that 1 to 2% (10 to 20 million) of the Indian population suffer from major mental disorders, and around 5% (50 million) suffer from minor mental disorders.

Mental health services are provided mainly through psychiatric hospitals, psychiatric nursing homes, observation wards, day centers, inpatient treatment in general hospitals, ambulatory treatment facilities, and other facilities such as halfway homes.

There are 37 government-run psychiatric hospitals in India, most of which are managed by state governments. These facilities have a total capacity of 18000 inpatients; almost half of available beds are occupied by long stay patients. In any event, mental health care is often out of reach for the roughly one third of the population who lives below the poverty line.

Three laws directly address mental health: The Narcotic Drugs and Psychotropic Substances Act, 1985; Mental Health Act, 1987; and the Persons with Disability Act, 1995. In addition, the National Health Policy of 2002 specifies the inclusion of mental health in general health services. The common selected facts about mental disorders are given in Table 1.1.

Table 1.1: Selected facts about mental disorders

- 450 million people worldwide are suffering from one or another mental illness. Many people suffer at once by several types of mental illness.
- Mental disorders occupy four of the ten positions in the list of the main causes of incapacity to work in developed countries (major depression, bipolar disorder, schizophrenia and obsessive-compulsive disorder).
- The most common mental disorders—the so-called anxiety disorders: panic disorder, obsessive-compulsive disorder, post-traumatic stress disorder and various phobias.
- 90% of people who commit suicide have depression or another diagnosable mental illness or are in drug or alcohol addiction.
- In some countries, deaths due to suicide exceed deaths from AIDS and some cancers.
- Men die from suicide four times more than women, although women are making three times more attempts to commit suicide.
- Suicide—the third leading cause of death among people aged 15–24 years.
- Attention deficit and hyperactivity disorder affects approximately every six months, 4.1% of children and adolescents from 9 to 17 years. Boys suffer from it 2–3 times more often than girls.
- Approximately 10% of patients with memory loss or other signs of dementia actually suffer from reversible diseases such as metabolic disorders, depression, intoxication or vitamin deficiency.
- Almost at 90% of people with Alzheimer's disease are observed depressive syndromes (25%—severe depression).
- The incidence of Alzheimer's disease in the age group over 65 years grows to twice every five years.
- One of 33 children and one of eight teenagers are affected of depression.
- Women suffer from depression almost twice as often as men.
- PMS suffer from up to 75% of women of reproductive age. In 60% of women with severe PMS, there are mental illnesses.
- Premenstrual dysphoria—is a severe form of PMS that affects 8% of women.

DEFINITION

Mental health: The capacity of an individual to form harmonious relationships with others and to participate in, or contribute contribute constructively to, changes in the social environment (WHO).

Mental health nursing: "A specialty nursing practice focusing on the *identification of mental health issues, prevention of mental health problems, and the care and treatment of persons with psychiatric disorders*."—The American Psychiatric Nurses Association

The scope of psychiatric nurses may be in general psychiatry care and specialized areas like child-adolescent mental health nursing, geriatric-psychiatric nursing, forensics, or substance-abuse.

CRITERIA FOR GOOD MENTAL HEALTH

There are six criteria of "the mentally healthy individual" proposed by Dr Marie Jahoda in her monograph, Current Concepts of Positive Mental Health:
1. He is self-reliant, self-confident and self-accepting.
2. His degree of self-actualization is such that his motivational processes can be characterized as growth motivation rather than need motivation.
3. He can resist stress, has a unifying outlook on life, and his psychic forces are in flexible balance; that is, he shows a relatively good integration of the personality.
4. He is autonomous (rather than, in Riesman's terms, either "adjusted" on the one hand or "anomic" on the other). He maintains a stable set of internal standards for his actions, so that he is relatively independent of social influences.
5. He is able to perceive the world and other persons with relative freedom from the distortions that may originate in his own needs. Related to this perception of reality is empathy, or social sensitivity, by virtue of which he will treat the inner life of others as a matter worthy of his concern.
6. He is adapted to his environment, displaying a creative capacity for love, work, and play.

CAUSES OF MENTAL DISORDERS

Biological Factors

Biochemical: Some mental illnesses have been linked to an abnormal balance of special chemicals in the brain called neurotransmitters. Neurotransmitters help nerve cells in the brain communicate with each other. If these chemicals are out of balance or are not working properly, messages may not make it through the brain correctly, leading to symptoms of mental illness.

Genetics (heredity): Many mental illnesses run in families, suggesting that people who have a family member with a mental illness are more likely to develop a mental illness. Susceptibility is passed on in families through genes.

Infections: Certain infections have been linked to brain damage and the development of mental illness or the worsening of its symptoms.

Brain defects or injury: Defects in or injury to certain areas of the brain have also been linked to some mental illnesses.

Prenatal damage: Some evidence suggests that a disruption of early fetal brain development or trauma that occurs at the time of birth—for example, loss of oxygen to the brain—may be a factor in the development of certain conditions, such as autism.

Substance abuse: Long-term substance abuse, in particular, has been linked to anxiety, depression, and paranoia.

Other factors: Poor nutrition and exposure to toxins, such as lead, may play a role in the development of mental illnesses.

Psychological Factors

- Severe psychological trauma suffered as a child, such as emotional, physical, or sexual abuse
- An important early loss, such as the loss of a parent
- Neglect
- Poor ability to relate to others.

Environmental Factors

- Death or divorce
- A dysfunctional family life
- Living in poverty
- Feelings of inadequacy, low self-esteem, anxiety, anger, or loneliness
- Changing jobs or schools
- Social or cultural expectations (for example, a society that associates beauty with thinness can be a factor in the development of eating disorders).
- Substance abuse by the person or the person's parents.

CLASSIFICATION OF MENTAL DISORDERS

International Statistical Classification of Diseases and Related Health Problems

The International Statistical Classification of Diseases and Related Health Problems 10th Revision (ICD-10) is a coding of diseases and signs, symptoms, abnormal findings, complaints, social circumstances and external causes of injury or diseases, as classified by the World Health Organization (WHO). Chapter V is discussing psychaitric problem as Mental and behavioral disorders and coded them F00 to F99.

F00-F99 Mental and behavioral disorders

F00–F09	Organic, including symptomatic, mental disorders
F10–F19	Mental and behavioral disorders duo to psychoactive substance use
F20–F29	Schizophrenia, schizotypal and delusional disorders
F30–F39	Mood (affective) disorders
F40–F48	Neurotic, stress related and somatoform disorders
F50–F59	Behavioral syndromes associated with physiological disturbances and physical factors
F60–F69	Disorders of adult personality and behavior
F70–F79	Mental retardation
F80–F89	Disorders of psychological development
F90–F98	Behavioral and emotional disorders with onset usually occurring in childhood and adolescence
F99	Unspecified mental disorders.

Diagnostic and Statistical Manual of Mental Disorders, Fourth Edition (DSM-IV)

Psychiatric Diagnoses are categorized by the Diagnostic and Statistical Manual of Mental Disorders, 4th Edition. Better known as the DSM-IV, the manual is published by the American Psychiatric Association and covers all mental health disorders for both children and adults. It also lists known causes of these disorders, statistics in terms of gender, age at onset, and prognosis as well as some research concerning the optimal treatment approaches.

It assesses five dimensions as described below:

Axis I: Clinical Syndromes
- This is what we typically think of as the diagnosis (e.g. depression, schizophrenia, social phobia).

Axis II: Developmental Disorders and Personality Disorders
- Developmental disorders include autism and mental retardation, disorders which are typically first evident in childhood
- Personality disorders are clinical syndromes which have a more long lasting symptoms and encompass the individual's way of interacting with the world. They include paranoid, antisocial, and borderline personality disorders.

Axis III: Physical Conditions which play a role in the development, continuance, or exacerbation of Axis I and II Disorders
- Physical conditions such as brain injury or HIV/AIDS that can result in symptoms of mental illness are included here.

Axis IV: Severity of Psychosocial Stressors
- Events in a persons life, such as death of a loved one, starting a new job, college, unemployment, and even marriage can impact the disorders listed in Axis I and II. These events are both listed and rated for this axis.

Axis V: Highest Level of Functioning
- On the final axis, the clinician rates the person's level of functioning both at the present time and the highest level within the previous year. This helps the clinician understand how the above four axes are affecting the person and what type of changes could be expected.

Indian Classification of Mental Disorder
Psychosis:
1. Functional psychosis, e.g. schizophrenia
2. Affective psychosis, e.g. mania and depression
3. Organic psychosis, e.g. delirium and dementia

Neurosis:
1. Anxiety
2. Depression
3. Hysteria
4. Obsessive compulsive disorder
5. Phobia

Special disorder:
1. Childhood mental disorder
2. Personality disorder
3. Psychoactive substance use disorder
4. Psychophysiological disorder
5. Mental retardation.

PRINCIPLES OF MENTAL HEALTH NURSING
- Allow client opportunity to set own pace in working with problems.
- Nursing interventions should center on the client as a person, not on control of the symptoms. Symptoms are important, but not as important as the person having them.
- Recognize your own feelings toward clients and deal with them.
- Go to the client who needs help the most.
- Do not allow a situation to develop or continue in which a client becomes the focus of attention in a negative manner.
- If client behavior is bizarre, base your decision to intervene on whether the client is endangering self or others.
- Ask for help—do not try to be a hero when dealing with a client who is out of control!
- Avoid highly competitive activities, that is, having one winner and a room full of losers.
- Make frequent contact with clients—it lets them know they are worth your time and effort.
- Remember to assess the physical needs of your client.

- Have patience! Move at the client's pace and ability.
- Suggesting, requesting, or asking works better than commanding.
- Therapeutic thinking is not thinking about or for, but with the client.
- Be honest, so the client can rely on you.
- Make reality interesting enough that the client prefers it to his or her fantasy.
- Compliment, reassure, and model appropriate behavior.

THE INTERDISCIPLINARY TREATMENT TEAM

Psychiatrist

Credentials: Medical degree with residency in psychiatry and license to practice medicine.

Responsibilities: Serves as the leader of the team. Responsible for diagnosis and treatment of mental disorders. Performs psychotherapy; prescribes medication and other somatic therapies.

Clinical Psychologist

Credentials: Doctorate in clinical psychology with 2–3 years internship supervised by a licensed clinical psychologist. State license is required for practice.

Responsibilities: Conducts individual, group and family therapy. Administers, interprets and evaluates psychological tests that can assist in the diagnostic process.

Psychiatric Clinical Nurse Specialist

Credentials: Registered nurse with a minimum of a master's degree in psychiatric nursing. Some institutions require certification by national credentialing association.

Responsibilities: Conducts individual, group and family therapy. Presents educational programs for nursing staff. Provides consultation services to nurses who require assistance in the planning and implementation of the care for individual clients.

Psychiatric Nurse

Credentials: Registered nurse with hospital diploma, associate degree or baccalaureate degree. Some psychiatric nurses have national certification.

Responsibilities: Provides ongoing assessment of client condition, both mentally and physically. Manages the therapeutic milieu on a 24 hours basis. Administers medications. Assists clients with all therapeutic activities as required. Focus is on one-to-one relationship development.

Mental Health Technician (Psychiatric Aide or Assistant or Psychiatric technician)

Credentials: Varies from state to state. Requirements include high school education, with additional vocational education or on the job training. Some hospitals hire individuals with baccalaureate degree in psychology in this capacity. Some states require a licensure examination to practice.

Responsibilities: Functions under the supervision of the psychiatric nurse. Provides assistance to the clients in the fulfillment of their activities of daily living. Assists activity therapists as required in conducting their groups. May also participate in one-to-one relationship development.

Psychiatric Social Worker

Credentials: Minimum of master's degree in social work. Some states require additional supervision and subsequent licensure by examination.

Responsibilities: Conducts individual, group and family therapy. Is concerned with client's social needs such as placement, financial support and community requirements. Conducts in depth psychosocial history on which the needs assessments is based. Works with client and family to ensure that requirements for discharge are fulfilled and needs can be met by appropriate community resources.

Occupational Therapist

Credentials: Baccalaureate or master's degree in occupational therapy.

Responsibilities: Work with clients to help to develop independence in performance of activities of daily living. Focus is on rehabilitation and vocational training in which clients learn to be productive, thereby enhancing self-esteem. Creative activities and therapeutic relationship skills are used.

Recreational Therapist

Credentials: Baccalaureate or master's degree in recreational therapy.

Responsibilities: Use recreational activities to promote clients to redirect their thinking or to rechannel their destructive energy in an appropriate manner. Clients learn skills that can be used during leisure time and during times of stress following discharge from treatment.

Music Therapist

Credentials: Graduate degree with specialty in music therapy.

Responsibilities: Encourages clients in self-expression through music. Clients listen to music, play instruments, sing, dance and compose songs that help them get in touch with feelings and emotions that they may not be able to experience in any other way.

Art Therapist

Credentials: Graduate degree with specialty in art therapy.

Responsibilities: Uses the client's creative abilities to encourage the expression of emotions and feelings through artwork. Helps client to analyze their own work in an effort to recognize and resolve underlying conflict.

Psyhcodramatist

Credentials: Graduate degree in psychology, social work, nursing or medicine with additional training in group therapy and specialty preparation to become Psyhcodramatist.
Responsibilities: Directs the clients in the creation of a drama that portrays real life situations. Individuals select problems they wish to enact, and other clients play the roles of significant others in the situations. Some clients are able to act out problems that they are unable to work through in a more traditional manner.

Dietitian

Credentials: Baccalaureate or master's degree with specialty in dietetics.
Responsibilities: Plans nutritious meals for all clients. Works on consulting basis for clients with specific eating disorders such as anorexia nervosa, bulimia nervosa, obesity and pica.

Chaplain

Credentials: College degree with advanced education in theology, seminary or rabbinical studies.
Responsibilities: Assess, identifies and attends to the spiritual needs of clients and their family members. Provides spiritual support and comfort as requested by client or family. May provide counseling if educational background includes this type of preparation.

PREVENTIVE PSYCHIATRY

It is defined as preventing mental illness, promoting mental health, proper diagnosis and treatment of mental illness and rehabilitate of patient to avoid disable and reoccurrence of illness.
Concepts of preventive psychiatry:
1. Primary prevention
2. Secondary prevention
3. Tertiary prevention.

Primary Prevention

Primary prevention aims at promotion of mental health and prevention of mental disorder, i.e. reduction of occurrence of new cases of mental disorders. The community mental health nurse has a significant role in the primary prevention. Promotion of mental health can be done by nurse by educating the members of the community on principles of mental health and mental hygiene by providing them the healthy coping mechanism in handling day by day stresses in life, etc.

Secondary Prevention

It focus on early identification and effective treatment for those suffering with mental disorders.

Tertiary Prevention

It aims to reduce the rate of disabilities duo to longer duration of suffering from mental disorder. It aims to helps the patient in the readjustment with the family and community from where he comes through rehabilitation program.

COMMUNITY FACILITIES AVAILABLE IN INDIA

Varied community facilities are available to provide mental health care for total population.

Day care centers: The client will receive the treatment and services during the day time. It is one of the methods under partial hospitalization.

Group homes: Nearly 15–20 recovered clients with significant mental illness will be placed in a home. They will live like a society, provides moral, emotional and social support to each other.

Quarter way home: This will be within the hospital but no regular service of the hospital staff will be available. Clients will carryout the activities.

Halfway homes: They offer a variety of therapies, facilities, transition between the hospital and independent living where the person is without the benefit of therapy except for weekly counseling sessions or maintenance drug therapy.

Foster homes: A household in which an orphaned or delinquent child is placed

Sheltered workshop: A workplace that provides a supportive environment where physically or mentally challenged persons can acquire job skills and vocational experience and they can earn wages but are free from the competitive stress of the usual job.

Mental health emergency care:

Hotline: A telephone line that gives quick and direct access to the mental health professionals to obtain information or help in case of an emergency.

Walk in clinic: It is a type of clinic, where 24 hours emergency diagnostic and therapeutic services will be provided.

Home visits: Community mental health team individually conducts domiciliary visits and provides care to the needy people at their door step.

Self-help groups: It is a group of individuals sharing a similar problem, who meet regularly to exchange information and to give and receive psychological support. Such groups run by the members themselves rather than by professionals.

Suicide prevention centers: These centers are helpful in identifying the risky population and assisting them in supportive services.

Chapter 2

Conceptual Models

PERSONALITY

"Personality" can be defined as a dynamic and organized set of characteristics possessed by a person that uniquely influences his or her cognitions, motivations and behaviors in various situations.

The word "personality" originates from the Latin *persona*, which means mask. Significantly, in the theater of the ancient Latin-speaking world, the mask was not used as a plot device to *disguise* the identity of a character, but rather was a convention employed to represent or *typify* that character. Personality may also refer to the patterns of thoughts, feelings and behaviors consistently exhibited by an individual over time that strongly influence our expectations, self-perceptions, values and attitudes, and predicts our reactions to people, problems and stress.

Types of Personality

People can be either extroverts or introverts, depending on the direction of their activity; thinking, feeling, sensing, intuitive, according to their own information pathways; judging or perceiving, depending on the method in which they process received information.

Extroverts vs Introverts

Extroverts are directed towards the objective world whereas Introverts are directed towards the subjective world. The most common differences between Extroverts and Introverts are given in Table 2.1:

Table 2.1: Differences between extroverts and introverts	
Extroverts	**Introverts**
• Are interested in what is happening around them • Are open and often talkative • Compare their own opinions with the opinions of others • Like action and initiative • Easily make new friends or adapt to a new group • Say what they think • Are interested in new people • Easily break unwanted relations	• Are interested in their own thoughts and feelings • Need to have own territory • Often appear reserved, quiet and thoughtful • Usually do not have many friends • Have difficulties in making new contacts • Like concentration and quiet • Do not like unexpected visits and therefore do not make them • Work well alone

Sensing vs Intuition

Sensing is an ability to deal with information on the basis of its physical qualities and its affection by other information. Intuition is an ability to deal with the information on the basis of its hidden potential and its possible existence. The most common differences between Sensing and Intuitive types are given in Table 2.2.

Table 2.2: Differences between sensing and intuitive types	
Sensing types	**Intuitive types**
• See everyone and sense everything • Live in the here and now • Quickly adapt to any situation • Like pleasures based on physical sensation • Are practical and active • Are realistic and self-confident	• Are mostly in the past or in the future • Worry about the future more than the present • Are interested in everything new and unusual • Do not like routine • Are attracted more to the theory than the practice • Often have doubts

Thinking vs Feeling

Thinking is an ability to deal with information on the basis of its structure and its function. Feeling is an ability to deal with information on the basis of its initial energetic condition and its interactions. The most common differences between Thinking and Feeling type are given in Table 2.3.

Table 2.3: Differences between thinking and feeling type	
Thinking types	**Feeling types**
• Are interested in systems, structures, patterns • Expose everything to logical analysis • Are relatively cold and unemotional • Evaluate things by intellect and right or wrong • Have difficulties talking about feelings • Do not like to clear up arguments or quarrels	• Are interested in people and their feelings • Easily pass their own moods to others • Pay great attention to love and passion • Evaluate things by ethics and good or bad • Can be touchy or use emotional manipulation • Often give compliments to please people

Perceiving vs Judging

Perceiving types are motivated into activity by the changes in a situation. Judging types are motivated into activity by their decisions resulting from the changes in a situation. The most common differences between Perceiving and Judging types are given in Table 2.4.

FREUD THEORY

The **conscious mind** is what you are aware of at any particular moment, your present perceptions, memories, thoughts, fantasies, feelings, what have you.

Table 2.4: Differences between perceiving and judging type

Perceiving types	Judging types
• Act impulsively following the situation • Can start many things at once without finishing them properly • Prefer to have freedom from obligations • Are curious and like a fresh look at things • Work productivity depends on their mood • Often act without any preparation	• Do not like to leave unanswered questions • Plan work ahead and tend to finish it • Do not like to change their decisions • Have relatively stable workability • Easily follow rules and discipline

Working closely with the conscious mind is what Freud called the **preconscious,** what we might today call "available memory;" anything that can easily be made conscious, the memories you are not at the moment thinking about but can readily bring to mind.

The largest part by far is the **unconscious**. It includes all the things that are not easily available to awareness, including many things that have their origins there, such as our drives or instincts, and things that are put there because we can't bear to look at them, such as the memories and emotions associated with trauma.

Freudian psychological reality begins with the world, full of objects. Among them is a very special object, the organism. The organism is special in that it acts to survive and reproduce, and it is guided toward those ends by its needs—hunger, thirst, the avoidance of pain, and sex.

A part—a very important part—of the organism is the nervous system, which has as one of its characteristics a sensitivity to the organism's needs. At birth, that nervous system is little more than that of any other animal, an "it" or **id**. The nervous system, as id, translates the organism's needs into motivational forces called, in German, **Triebe**, which has been translated as **instincts** or **drives**. Freud also called them **wishes**. This translation from need to wish is called the **primary process**.

The id works in keeping with the **pleasure principle**, which can be understood as a demand to take care of needs immediately. Just picture the hungry infant, screaming itself blue. It does not "know" what it wants in any adult sense; it just knows that it wants it and it wants it now. The infant, in the Freudian view, is pure, or nearly pure id. And the id is nothing if not the psychic representative of biology.

Unfortunately, although a wish for food, such as the image of a juicy steak, might be enough to satisfy the id, it is not enough to satisfy the organism. The need only gets stronger, and the wishes just keep coming. You may have noticed that, when you have not satisfied some need, such as the need for food, it begins to demand more and more of your attention, until there comes a point where you can not think of anything else. This is the wish or drive breaking into consciousness.

Luckily for the organism, there is that small portion of the mind we discussed before, the conscious, that is hooked up to the world through the senses. Around this little bit of consciousness, during the first year of a child's life, some of the

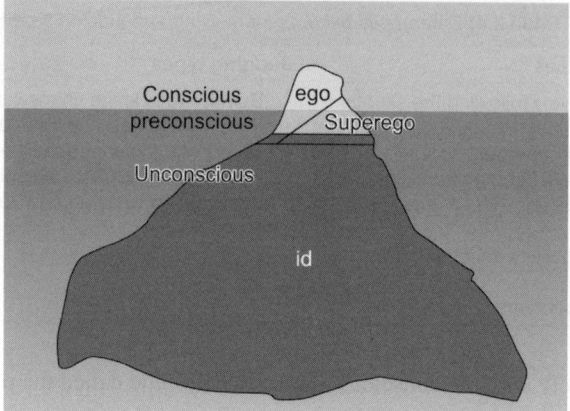

Figure 2.1: The id, the ego, and the superego

"it" becomes "I," some of the id becomes ego. The **ego** relates the organism to reality by means of its consciousness, and it searches for objects to satisfy the wishes that id creates to represent the organisms needs. This problem-solving activity is called the **secondary process**.

The ego, unlike the id, functions according to the reality principle, which says "take care of a need as soon as an appropriate object is found." It represents reality and, to a considerable extent, reason.

However, as the ego struggles to keep the id (and, ultimately, the organism) happy, it meets with obstacles in the world. It occasionally meets with objects that actually assist it in attaining its goals. And it keeps a record of these obstacles and aides. In particular, it keeps track of the rewards and punishments meted out by two of the most influential objects in the world of the child—mom and dad. This record of things to avoid and strategies to take becomes the superego. It is not completed until about seven years of age. In some people, it never is completed.

There are two aspects to the superego: One is the **conscience**, which is an internalization of punishments and warnings. The other is called the **ego ideal**. It derives from rewards and positive models presented to the child. The conscience and ego ideal communicate their requirements to the ego with feelings like pride, shame and guilt. This theory well understood by the schematic diagram (Fig. 2.1).

PSYCHOSEXUAL STAGE THEORY

The oral stage lasts from birth to about 18 months. The focus of pleasure is, of course, the mouth. Sucking and biting are favorite activities.

The anal stage lasts from about 18 months to three or four years old. The focus of pleasure is the anus. Holding it in and letting it go are greatly enjoyed.

The phallic stage lasts from three or four to five, six, or seven years old. The focus of pleasure is the genitalia. Masturbation is common.

The latent stage lasts from five, six, or seven to puberty, that is, somewhere around 12 years old. During this stage, Freud believed that the sexual impulse

was suppressed in the service of learning. I must note that, while most children seem to be fairly calm, sexually, during their grammar school years, perhaps up to a quarter of them are quite busy masturbating and playing "doctor." In Freud's repressive era, these children were, at least, quieter than their modern counterparts.

The genital stage begins at puberty, and represents the resurgence of the sex drive in adolescence, and the more specific focusing of pleasure in sexual intercourse. Freud felt that masturbation, oral sex, homosexuality, and many other things we find acceptable in adulthood today, were immature.

ERIK ERIKSON'S 8 STAGES OF PSYCHOSOCIAL DEVELOPMENT

Stage 1—Basic Trust vs Mistrust

- Developing trust is the first task of the ego, and it is never complete.
- The child will let mother out of sight without anxiety and rage because she has become an inner certainty as well as an outer predictability.
- The balance of trust with mistrust depends largely on the quality of maternal relationship.

Stage 2—Autonomy vs Shame and Doubt

- If denied autonomy, the child will turn against him/herself urges to manipulate and discriminate.
- Shame develops with the child's self-consciousness.
- Doubt has to do with having a front and back—a "behind" subject to its own rules. Left over doubt may become paranoia.
- The sense of autonomy fostered in the child and modified as life progresses serves the preservation in economic and political life of a sense of justice.

Stage 3—Initiative vs Guilt

- Initiative adds to autonomy the quality of undertaking, planning, and attacking a task for the sake of being active and on the move.
- The child feels guilt over the goals contemplated and the acts initiated in exuberant enjoyment of new locomoter and mental powers.
- The castration complex occuring in this stage is due to the child's erotic fantasies.
- A residual conflict over initiative may be expressed as hysterical denial, which may cause the repression of the wish or the abrogation of the child's ego: Paralysis and inhibition, or overcompensation and showing off.
- The Oedipal stage results not only in oppressive establishment of a moral sense restricting the horizon of the permissible, but also sets the direction towards the possible and the tangible which permits dreams of early childhood to be attached to goals of an active adult life.

After Stage 3, one may use the whole repetoire of previous modalities, modes, and zones for industrious, identity-maintaining, intimate, legacy-producing, dispair-countering purposes.

Stage 4—Industry vs Inferiority

- To bring a productive situation to completion is an aim which gradually supersedes the whims and wishes of play.
- The fundamentals of technology are developed.
- To lose the hope of such "industrious" association may pull the child back to the more isolated, less conscious familial rivalry of the Oedipal time.
- The child can become a conformist and thoughtless slave whom others exploit.

Stage 5—Identity vs Role Confusion (or Diffusion)

- The adolescent is newly concerned with how they appear to others.
- Ego identity is the accrued confidence that the inner sameness and continuity prepared in the past are matched by the sameness and continuity of one's meaning for others, as evidenced in the promise of a career.
- The inability to settle on a school or occupational identity is disturbing.

Stage 6—Intimacy vs Isolation

- Body and ego must be masters of organ modes and of the other nuclear conflicts in order to face the fear of ego loss in situations which call for self-abandon.
- The avoidance of these experiences leads to isolation and self-absorption.
- The counterpart of intimacy is distantiation, which is the readiness to isolate and destroy forces and people whose essence seems dangerous to one's own.
- Now true genitality can fully develop.
- The danger at this stage is isolation which can lead to sever character problems.

Erikson's listed criteria for "genital utopia" illustrate his insistence on the role of many modes and modalities in harmony: (i) mutuality of orgasm, (ii) with a loved partner, (iii) of opposite sex, (iv) with whom one is willing and able to share a trust, and, (v) with whom one is willing and able to regulate the cycles of work, procreation, and recreation, (vi) so as to secure to the offspring all the stages of satisfactory development.

Stage 7—Generativity vs Stagnation

- Generativity is the concern in establishing and guiding the next generation.
- Simply having or wanting children does not achieve generativity.
- Socially-valued work and disciples are also expressions of generativity.

Stage 8—Ego Integrity vs Despair

- Ego integrity is the ego's accumulated assurance of its capacity for order and meaning.
- Despair is signified by a fear of one's own death, as well as the loss of self-sufficiency, and of loved partners and friends.
- Healthy children, Erikson tells us, would not fear life if their elders have integrity enough not to fear death.

KOHLBERG'S THEORY OF MORAL DEVELOPMENT

Moral development is the development of a sense of right and wrong.
- There are three levels to Kohlberg's theory of moral development (Table 2.5).
- The premoral level occurs during early childhood, where the actions of a child are influenced more by fear than by what is right or wrong.
- An amoral person is a person who does not know the difference between right and wrong, and does not feel guilt for doing the wrong thing.
- The conventional level begins during late childhood and extends until the end of adolescence. Most adults will remain in this level.
- In the conventional level, we regard something to be right because we have been told it is right. As a result, we do not question it very much and go along with what we are told.
- The principled level is the highest level of Kohlberg's theory of moral development, and is characterized by an individual's ability to think for themselves by logically deciding what is right or wrong.

Table 2.5: Moral developmental theory

Premoral Level	
Stage 1: Punishment-Avoidance and obedience	Make moral decisions strictly on the basis of self-interests. Disobey rules if can do so without getting caught.
Stage 2: Exchange of favors	Recognize that others have needs, but make satisfaction of own needs a higher priority
Conventional Level	
Stage 3: Good boy/good girl	Make decisions on the basis of what will please others. Concerned about maintaining interpersonal relations
Stage 4: Law and order	Look to society as a while for guidelines about behavior. Think rules as inflexible, unchangeable.
Principled Level	
Stage 5: Social contract	Recognize that rules are social agreements that can be changed when necessary
Stage 6: Universal ethical principle	Adhere to a small number of abstract principles that transcend specific, concrete rules. Answer to an inner conscience.

PEPLAU'S INTERPERSONAL THEORY

Peplau's theory focuses on the interpersonal processes and therapeutic relationship that develops between the nurse and client. The interpersonal focus of Peplau's theory requires that the nurse attend to the interpersonal processes that occur between the nurse and client. Interpersonal process is maturing force for personality. Interpersonal processes include the nurse–client relationship, communication, pattern integration and the roles of the nurse. Psychodynamic nursing is being able to understand one's own behavior to help others identify felt difficulties and to apply principles of human relations to the problems that arise at

all levels of experience. This theory stressed the importance of nurses' ability to understand own behavior to help others identify perceived difficulties.

The four Phases of Nurse-Patient Relationships are:

1. Orientation
During this phase, the individual has a *felt need* and seeks professional assistance. The nurse helps the individual to recognize and understand his/her problem and determine the need for help.

2. Identification
The patient identifies with those who can help him/her. The nurse permits exploration of feelings to aid the patient in undergoing illness as an experience that reorients feelings and strengthens positive forces in the personality and provides needed satisfaction.

3. Exploitation
During this phase, the patient attempts to derive full value from what he/she are offered through the relationship. The nurse can project new goals to be achieved through personal effort and power shifts from the nurse to the patient as the patient delays gratification to achieve the newly formed goals.

4. Resolution
The patient gradually puts aside old goals and adopts new goals. This is a process in which the patient frees himself from identification with the nurse.

PIAGET'S THEORY OF COGNITIVE DEVELOPMENT

The most well-known and influential theory of cognitive development is that of Swiss psychologist Jean Piaget (1896–1980).

Piaget termed assimilation and accommodation. Assimilation refers to the process of taking in new information by incorporating it into an existing schema. In other words, people assimilate new experiences by relating them to things they already know. On the other hand, accommodation is what happens when the schema itself changes to accommodate new knowledge. According to Piaget, cognitive development involves an ongoing attempt to achieve a balance between assimilation and accommodation that he termed equilibration.

At the center of Piaget's theory is the principle that cognitive development occurs in a series of four distinct, universal stages, each characterized by increasingly sophisticated and abstract levels of thought. These stages always occur in the same order, and each builds on what was learned in the previous stage. They are as follows:
- Sensorimotor stage (infancy): In this period, which has six sub-stages, intelligence is demonstrated through motor activity without the use of symbols. Knowledge of the world is limited, but developing, because it is based on physical interactions and experiences. Children acquire object permanence at about seven months of age (memory). Physical development (mobility)

allows the child to begin developing new intellectual abilities. Some symbolic (language) abilities are developed at the end of this stage.

- Preoperational stage (toddlerhood and early childhood): In this period, which has two sub-stages, intelligence is demonstrated through the use of symbols, language use matures, and memory and imagination are developed, but thinking is done in a non-logical, non-reversible manner. Egocentric thinking predominates.
- Concrete operational stage (elementary and early adolescence): In this stage, characterized by seven types of conservation (number, length, liquid, mass, weight, area, and volume), intelligence is demonstrated through logical and systematic manipulation of symbols related to concrete objects. Operational thinking develops (mental actions that are reversible). Egocentric thought diminishes.
- Formal operational stage (adolescence and adulthood): In this stage, intelligence is demonstrated through the logical use of symbols related to abstract concepts. Early in the period there is a return to egocentric thought. Only 35% of high school graduates in industrialized countries obtain formal operations; many people do not think formally during adulthood.

Chapter 3

Mental Health Assessment

HISTORY COLLECTION

It is the patients life story told to the clinician by the patient and if necessary from informed source to make a *correct diagnosis and formulate a specific and effective treatment plan.*

Purpose

- To describe the patients condition, family, development and environmental factors affecting his behavior
- To identify symptoms of illness, their development over time and the effect on the persons life
- To detect and understand the significance of factors that caused the illness
- Identify factors which will affect the management and outcome of the illness
- Identify psychiatric emergencies
- Plan and implement nursing interventions.

Components of History Collection

A. Sociodemographic data
- Name
- Age/sex
- Mother tongue
- Religion
- Occupation
- Marital status
- Education
- Socioeconomic status—high/middle/low
- Source of referral
- Address
- Informant—who, reliable/not; complete/not;

Date of interview
Date of admission
Bed no:

B. Chief complaints
Symptoms and duration in chronological order, for example:
- Decreased work output 15 days
- Decreased sleep 5 days
- Decreased appetite 3 days.

C. History of present illness
Onset
- Mode of onset
  - Abrupt (< 24 hours)
  - Acute (within 2 weeks)
  - Subacute (> 2 weeks)
  - Insidious (> 4 weeks)
- Course—episodic/continuous/fluctuations
- Precipitating factors
- Perpetuating factors

D. Past history
- Psychiatric history
  - Any psychiatric illness in the past, symptoms, duration, treatment taken—regular/not, response, specify each episode
- Medical history
  - Any head injury, convulsions, unconsciousness, diabetes mellitus, hypertension, HIV/AIDS, etc.

E. Family history
- Of similar illness
- Associated illness
- Medical illness
- Substance dependence
- Suicidal attempt/suicide
- Treatment taken and relief obtained.

F. Personal history
- Birth and early development
  - FTND/premature
  - Home/hospital delivery
  - APGAR'S score
    - any complications
  - Milestones—normal/not
  - Feeding, sleeping, playing, parents involvement with child
- Childhood history
  - Behavior
  - Schooling
  - Physical illness—epilepsy, meningitis, encephalitis
  - Any fears/phobias, nail biting, bed wetting thumb sucking
- Educational history:
  - Age at which began, level of education
  - Achievement
  - Problems encountered

- Puberty and menstrual history
  - Onset of puberty
  - Cycles—regular/not, PMS if any
  - Problems encountered
- Occupational history
  - Present occupation
  - Attitude towards colleagues/seniors/subordinates/working environment
  - Job satisfaction/hopes/chances of promotions/ambitions
  - Past jobs held
  - Reason for changes of job
  - Any memos/absenteeism, etc. in present job/past job
  - Stressors at job place
  - Occupational deterioration at present
- Sexual history and marital history:
  - Knowledge level
  - Any extramarital relationship
  - Present marital relationship
  - Use/abuse of alcohol/drugs, etc.

G. Pre-morbid personality:

- Temperament
- Interpersonal relationship/social relationship
- Use of leisure time, hobbies
- Predominant mood—bright/cheerful/worrying
- Character—attitude to self/others
- Religious beliefs and moral attitudes
- Fantasy life—day dreaming
- Habits—food fads, self-medication, etc.

MENTAL STATUS EXAMINATION (MSE)

Mental status examination is a standardized format in which the clinician records the psychiatric signs and symptoms present at the time of interview.

Objectives

1. To confirm the signs and symptoms narrated by patient and his relatives in history.
2. It provides an opportunity to observe patient and elicit and clarify symptoms.

Mental status examination is covered systematically under the following readings:

1. General appearance and behavior
2. Speech
3. Mood and affect
4. Thought
5. Perception

6. Cognition
7. Insight
8. Judgement.

General Appearance and Behavior

- General appearance
  - Physical characteristics
  - Apparent age
  - Cleanliness (peculiarities of) dressing
  - Grooming
- Level of consciousness—alert/lethargic
- Motor
  - Status—posture (erect, stooped) gait (shuffling, awkward)
  - Activity—over or under active, sterotype, graceful
  - Facial expression:
    - Verbal and nonverbal expressions
    - Worried, sad, happy, frightened, laughing, smiling, suspicious (facial expression control)
    - Alert, angry, afraid, tense
- Behavior
  - Indifferent, frank, embarrassed, irritable, angry, friendly, assaultive, dramatic, exhibitionistic
- Relationship to examiner
  - Cooperative/non-cooperative
  - Comfortable/uncomfortable
  - Guardedness/insecuredness
  - Altentive/neglected
  - Friendliness/believeness.

Speech

- Description
  - Soft, loud, stuttering, hesistant, mutism
- Speed and quantity
  - Fast/delay in answering
  - Relationship with motor activity
  - Volume and tone (increased/decreased).

Emotion

- Mood
  - The subjective statement of his feeling state
- Affect
  - Observing patient's appearance and behavior (including verbal and nonverbal)

- Emotional display in association with situation
- Exhibition cheerfulness, sarcastic, hostile, depression, tensed, dull, apathetic.

Perceptions

- Illusion
  - Misperceptions of external stimuli
- Hallucinations
  - Auditory
  - Visual
  - Olfactory
  - Gustatory
  - Tactied.

Thoughts

- Content
  - Spontaneous trends of thought toward particular topics and preoccupation with these topics can be noted.
  - Delusions of percecution, delusion of grandeur and somatic delusion due to severe illness, for example, cancer.
- Progression
  - Associations, circumstantiality, blocking and flight of ideas.

Cognition

- Consiousness
  - Whether conscious, confusion, clouding, delirium, stupor, coma to be assessed
- Orientation
  - Time
  - Place
  - Person
  - Self
- Attention
  - Digit span test, digit forward and backward test to be done.
- Concentration
  - In the patient easily distractible or able to concentrate to be tested by giving simple mathematical problems.
- Memory
  - Immediate
  - Recent
  - Remote
- Intellecent
  - General information
  - Calculation
  - Reasoning and judgement
  - Proverb interpretation
  - Similarties.

Insight
- Realization of (patients) symptoms, current situation, understanding of need of help.

Judgement
- Social judgement
  - It is observed during the hospital stay and during the interview session. It includes the evaluation of personal judgement.
- Test judgement
  - It is assessed by asking the patient what he would do in certain test situation like a house on fire or man lying on the road or a seated stamped addressed envelop lying on a street.

Judgement is rated as good/intact/normal.

MINI MENTAL STATE EXAMINATION (MMSE)

Mini mental state examination or Folstein test is a brief 30 point questionnaire test that is used to screen for cognitive impairment and dementia.

The MMSE test includes simple questions and problems in a number of areas and it is explained in Table 3.1.

Table 3.1: Mini mental status examination

Category possible	Points	Description
Orientation to time	5	What is the (year) (season) (date) (day) (month)?
Orientation to place	5	Where are we (state) (country) (city) (hospital) (floor)?
Registration	3	Name 3 objects: One second to say each. Then ask the patient all three after you have said them. Give one point for each correct answer. Repeat them until he learns all three (note number of trials).
Attention and calculation	5	Begin with 100 and count backwards by 7 (stop after five answers).
Recall	3	Ask for three objects repeated above. Give one point for each correct answer.
Language	2	Show a pencil and a watch and ask subject to name them.
Repetition	1	Speaking back a phrase.
Complex commands	3	Take a paper in your right hand; fold it in half and put it on the floor.
	1	Read the obey the following (show subject the written items).
	1	Close your eyes, write a sentence.
	1	Copy a design.

Interpretation

A greater than or equal to 25 points—normal
- 21–24 points—mild cognitive impairment
- 10–20 points—moderate cognitive impairment
- Below 9—severe cognitive impairment.

NEUROLOGICAL EXAMINATION

The neurological examination is divided into several components, each focusing on a different part of the nervous system:
- Mental status
- Cranial nerves
- Motor system
- Sensory system
- The deep tendon reflexes
- Coordination and the cerebellum
- Gait.

The exam requires skill, patience, and intelligence on the part of the physician, and cooperation from the patient. Incomplete or inaccurate exams can lead to incorrect diagnoses.

Mental Status

The mental status examination is a series of detailed but simple questions designed to test cognitive ability, including the patient's:
- State of consciousness (awareness and responsiveness to the environment and the senses)
- Appearance and general behavior
- Mood
- Content of thought, and
- Intellectual resources (orientation with reference to time, place, and person; comprehension; ability to pay attention; insight; memory; judgment; abstract reasoning power; speech and language function; and intellectual capacity).

The patient may be asked to remember objects that had been listed earlier in the course of the exam; repeat sentences; solve simple mathematical problems; copy a three-dimensional drawing; and draw a clock and place the numbers and hands appropriately. When speech and language are tested, the examiner listens to the character of the speech, the fluency (smoothness of speech), and the patient's ability to understand and carry out simple or complex commands, and to read and write.

In addition, to specific questions that make up the actual mental status exam, the neurologist obtains important information by observing the patient's general behavior during the examination.

Many neurological diseases, such as dementia, cause changes in intellectual status or emotional responsiveness, and specific personality features. These

changes and features can be detected during the mental status portion of the neurological exam.

The mental status exam is especially important when the other parts of the neurological exam reveal no abnormalities. Sometimes, slight changes in memory or other intellectual resources may be the only indication that something is wrong. Evaluating a person's intellectual capacity can also be helpful in determining a course of treatment and making a prognosis.

Cranial Nerves

Observation

- Ptosis (III)
- Facial Droop or Asymmetry (VII)
- Hoarse Voice (X)
- Articulation of Words (V, VII, X, XII)
- Abnormal Eye Position (III, IV, VI)
- Abnormal or Asymmetrical Pupils (II, III)

I. Olfactory
Not normally tested.

II. Optic
- Examine the optic fundi
- Test visual acuity
  - Allow the patient to use their glasses or contact lens if available. You are interested in the patient's best corrected vision.
  - Position the patient 20 feet in front of the Snellen eye chart (or hold a Rosenbaum pocket card at a 14 inch "reading" distance).
  - Have the patient cover one eye at a time with a card.
  - Ask the patient to read progressively smaller letters until they can go no further.
  - Record the smallest line the patient read successfully (20/20, 20/30, etc.)
  - Repeat with the other eye.
- Screen visual fields by confrontation
  - Stand two feet in front of the patient and have them look into your eyes.
  - Hold your hands about one foot away from the patient's ears, and wiggle a finger on one hand.
  - Ask the patient to indicate which side they see the finger move.
  - Repeat two or three times to test both temporal fields.

- If an abnormality is suspected, test the four quadrants of each eye while asking the patient to cover the opposite eye with a card.
- Test pupillary reactions to light
  - Dim the room lights as necessary.
  - Ask the patient to look into the distance.
  - Shine a bright light obliquely into each pupil in turn.
  - Look for both the direct (same eye) and consensual (other eye) reactions.
  - Record pupil size in mm and any asymmetry or irregularity.
  - If abnormal, proceed with the test for accommodation.
- Test pupillary reactions to accommodation
  - Hold your finger about 10 cm from the patient's nose.
  - Ask them to alternate looking into the distance and at your finger.
  - Observe the pupillary response in each eye.

III. Oculomotor
- Observe for ptosis
- Test extraocular movements
  - Stand or sit 3 to 6 feet in front of the patient.
  - Ask the patient to follow your finger with their eyes without moving their head.
  - Check gaze in the six cardinal directions using a cross or "H" pattern.
  - Pause during upward and lateral gaze to check for nystagmus.
  - Check convergence by moving your finger toward the bridge of the patient's nose.
- Test pupillary reactions to light.

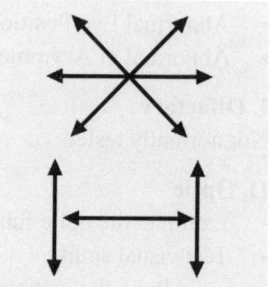

IV. Trochlear
Test extraocular movements (inward and down movement)

V. Trigeminal
- Test temporal and masseter muscle strength
  - Ask patient to both open their mouth and clench their teeth
  - Palpate the temporal and massetter muscles as they do this.
- Test the three divisions for pain sensation
  - Explain what you intend to do.
  - Use a suitable sharp object to test the forehead, cheeks, and jaw on both sides.
  - Substitute a blunt object occasionally and ask the patient to report "sharp" or "dull."
- If you find and abnormality then:
  - Test the three divisions for temperature sensation with a tuning fork heated or cooled by water.
  - Test the three divisions for sensation to light touch using a wisp of cotton.

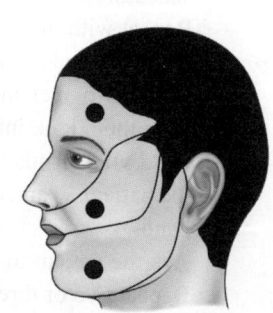

- Test the corneal reflex
  - Ask the patient to look up and away
  - From the other side, touch the cornea lightly with a fine wisp of cotton
  - Look for the normal blink reaction of **both** eyes
  - Repeat on the other side
  - Use of contact lens may decrease this response.

VI. Abducens
Test extraocular movements (lateral movement).

VII. Facial
- Observe for any facial droop or asymmetry
- Ask patient to do the following, note any lag, weakness, or asymmetry:
  - Raise eyebrows
  - Close both eyes to resistance
  - Smile
  - Frown
  - Show teeth
  - Puff out cheeks
- Test the corneal reflex

VIII. Acoustic
- Screen hearing
  - Face the patient and hold out your arms with your fingers near each ear
  - Rub your fingers together on one side while moving the fingers noiselessly on the other
  - Ask the patient to tell you when and on which side they hear the rubbing.
  - Increase intensity as needed and note any assymetry
  - If abnormal, proceed with the Weber and Rinne tests.
- Test for lateralization (Weber)
  - Use a 512 Hz or 1024 Hz tuning fork
  - Start the fork vibrating by tapping it on your opposite hand
  - Place the base of the tuning fork firmly on top of the patient's head
  - Ask the patient where the sound appears to be coming from (normally in the midline).
- Compare air and bone conduction (Rinne)
  - Use a 512 Hz or 1024 Hz tuning fork.
  - Start the fork vibrating by tapping it on your opposite hand.
  - Place the base of the tuning fork against the mastoid bone behind the ear.
  - When the patient no longer hears the sound, hold the end of the fork near the patient's ear (air conduction is normally greater than bone conduction).
- Vestibular function is not normally tested.

IX. Glossopharyngeal
See Vagus Nerve

X. Vagus
- Listen to the patient's voice, is it hoarse or nasal?
- Ask patient to swallow
- Ask patient to say "Ah"
  - Watch the movements of the soft palate and the pharynx.
- Test gag reflex (unconscious/uncooperative patient)
  - Stimulate the back of the throat on each side
  - It is normal to gag after each stimulus.

XI. Accessory
- From behind, look for atrophy or assymetry of the trapezius muscles
- Ask patient to shrug shoulders against resistance
- Ask patient to turn their head against resistance. Watch and palpate the sternomastoid muscle on the opposite side.

XII. Hypoglossal
- Listen to the articulation of the patient's words
- Observe the tongue as it lies in the mouth
- Ask patient to:
  - Protrude tongue
  - Move tongue from side to side.

Motor System

The motor system includes the brain and spinal cord motor pathways, and all the motor nerves and muscles throughout the body. Abnormalities in the motor system can often be detected by assessing muscle strength and tone and by looking for a variety of characteristic signs.

The patient is usually asked to undress, so the neurologist can see the muscles and look for atrophy (shrinkage), twitching, or abnormal movements. Tests are done to evaluate strength in all the major muscle groups.

Evaluating Babinski response is an important part of testing the motor system. The neurologist strokes or scratches, heel-to-toe, the outer side of the sole of the foot and in patients over the age of 2, the toes normally curl downward in response. If the toes fan upward, a brain or spinal cord injury is indicated. A number of neurological disorders can lead to Babinski response.

Sensory System

Sensation depends on impulses that occur as a result of stimulation of receptors located in the skin, muscles, tendons, and so on, and are sent along nerve fibers to the central nervous system (brain and spinal cord). The sensory exam is used to determine areas of abnormal sensation, the quality and type of sensation impairment, and the degree and extent of tissue involvement.

A sensory exam involves evaluating different types of sensation, including pain, temperature, pressure, and position. For example, pinpricks may be used to test the patient's response to pain and compare the response in different parts or opposite sides of the body. A cold or warm object may be used to test the sensation of temperature. To test position, patients may be asked to close their eyes and determine in which direction the examiner is moving a part of their body (e.g. big toe). Patients also may be asked to identify objects with their eyes closed or identify numbers or letters traced on their body.

The sensory exam should be repeated to provide accurate results. Responses may be affected by how alert, aware, and well-rested the patient is, so this part of the neurological exam is usually performed early in the course of testing.

Deep Tendon Reflexes

Reflexes are actions performed involuntarily in response to impulses sent to the central nervous system. Alterations in reflexes are often the first sign of neurological dysfunction. Observing reflexes is the most objective part of the neurological exam, since the reflexes are not under voluntary control and testing does not depend on the patient's cooperation, attitude, or awareness.

Hundreds of reflexes have been identified, but the neurological exam generally involves testing only the deep tendon reflexes. Deep tendon reflexes, also known as muscle stretch reflexes, are reflexes elicited in response to stimuli to tendons. Normally, when a specific area of the muscle tendon is tapped with a soft rubber hammer, the muscle fibers contract. Abnormal responses may indicate injury to the nervous system pathways that produce the deep tendon reflex.

Coordination and the Cerebellum

The cerebellum is the part of the brain that controls voluntary movement and motor coordination, including posture. Testing coordination provides clues about conditions that affect the cerebellum.

The neurologist may ask patients to move their finger from their nose to the neurologist's finger, going back and forth from nose to finger, touching the tip of each. Patients also may be asked to tap their fingers together quickly in a coordinated fashion or move their hands one on top of the other, back and forth, as smoothly as they can. Coordination in the lower limbs can be tested by asking patients to rub one heel up and down smoothly over the other shin.

Gait

Most of us take our ability to walk for granted. But as simple as it may seem, walking is a very intricate physiological process. How we walk—our gait—is influenced by a number of bodily mechanisms and nervous system reflexes. The body must be held erect; the limbs, head, and trunk must be held in the right position; the person must be oriented to the position of all body parts; parts of motor control involved with moving must be integrated; and so on.

Because walking depends on so many different parts of the nervous system, it can be affected by a variety of neurological disorders.

By observing gait, the neurologist can gather important clues about what might be wrong. The patient is usually asked to walk in different ways (e.g. heel-to-toe in a straight line, turning abruptly, walking on the toes, walking on the heels, running).

PSYCHOLOGICAL TESTS

Achievement and aptitude tests are usually seen in educational or employment settings, and they attempt to measure either how much you know about a certain topic (i.e. your achieved knowledge), such as mathematics or spelling, or how much of a capacity you have (i.e. *your aptitude*) to master material in a particular area, such as mechanical relationships.

Intelligence tests attempt to measure your intelligence—that is, your basic ability to understand the world around you, assimilate its functioning, and apply this knowledge to enhance the quality of your life. Or, as Alfred Whitehead said about intelligence, "it enables the individual to profit by error without being slaughtered by it." Intelligence, therefore, is a measure of a potential, not a measure of what you've learned (as in an achievement test), and so it is supposed to be independent of culture. The challenge is to design a test that can actually be culture-free; most intelligence tests fail in this area to some extent for one reason or another.

Neuropsychological tests attempt to measure deficits in cognitive functioning (i.e. your ability to think, speak, reason, etc.) that may result from some sort of brain damage, such as a stroke or a brain injury.

Occupational tests attempt to match your interests with the interests of persons in known careers. The logic here is that if the things that interest you in life match up with, say, the things that interest most school teachers, then you might make a good school teacher yourself.

Personality tests attempt to measure your basic personality style and are most used in research of forensic settings to help with clinical diagnoses. Two of the most well-known personality tests are:
- The Minnesota Multiphasic Personality Inventory (MMPI), or the revised MMPI-2, composed of several hundred "yes or no" questions, and
- The Rorschach (the "inkblot test"), composed of several cards of inkblots— you simply give a description of the images and feelings you experience in looking at the blots.

Specific clinical tests attempt to measure specific clinical matters, such as your current level of anxiety or depression.

Chapter 4

Therapeutic Relationship

COMMUNICATION

- A personal, interactive system; a series of ever-changing, ongoing transactions in the environment.

Therapeutic Communication

A meaningful relationship between the patient and professional helper. The patient-centered approach is influenced and directed by the professional.

Components of the Communication Process (or Model)

- **A sender or encoder**—person sending the message—can be verbal or nonverbal.
- **A receiver or decoder**—gets the message.
- **A message**—unit of information received.
- **Message variables**—verbal and nonverbal communication.
  - Verbal—is written and spoken–structural defects, malfunctioning due to disease, auditory and verbal impairments, sensory deprivation, overload or learning disabilities may affect or decrease accurate communication. Examples: A schizophrenic person, a stutterer, a mentally retarded or autistic person.
  - Voice pitch, voice quality (harsh, weak or strained), voice amplification (soft or loud), words, grammar and understanding are included in assessment.
  - Nonverbal—is gestures, facial expressions and dress and represents 65% of the communication. Examples of nonverbal behavior include: Crying, screaming, laughing, moaning, giggling and sighing, facial expression, body posture, gait, tone of voice and gestures.
  - Space and territory are forms of nonverbal communication as well. Personal space is the space preferred for interactions. Territory refers to implied space such as a patient's room or a specific seating arrangement.
  - Intrusion or violation of these areas can distract or distort communication.
- **Noise**—sound interference can impair accurate transmission.
- **Communication skills**—include being able to observe, listen, clarify and validate by both sender and receiver.
- **Setting**—where communication takes place.
- **Media**—refers to sensory channels that carry the message – hearing, sight, touch, taste and smell. Example: You get the message a patient needs pain

medication – you hear (hearing) complaints of pain, you see (sight) tears in their eyes, they grasp (touch) your arm in pain.
- **Feedback**—involves the continuous interpretation of response of the sender and receiver as messages are simultaneously encoded and decoded.
- **Environment**—are the internal and external influences affecting the communication process. External examples: room temperature, smells and lighting. Internal examples: Feeling cold, tired or experiencing pain.

Interpersonal Communication

- It is the most direct and pertinent form of communication because through this transaction needs are met.
- The main focus of interaction occurs at the interpersonal and group levels.
- There are three basic interpersonal styles of communicating:
  - Nonassertive or passive—letting others control behavior
  - Aggressive—threatening, blaming and hostile
  - Assertive—openly expressive, spontaneous, yet considerate of others.

Important Elements in Therapeutic Communication

- Empathy—which is a communication skill and behavior.
- Attending—being with the patient both in physical and psychological presence.
- Observing
- Listening.

Congruence between Verbal and Nonverbal Communication

There are two levels to every message—content and feeling — when content and feeling do not 'match' this is termed incongruent. Example: A patient with a sad facial expression and tear filled eyes, tells you he is fine. Or a husband says he is supportive of his wife's therapy but will be too busy to attend family sessions with her.

Barriers to Therapeutic Communication

- Lack of planning by the nurse.
- Poor data collection.
- Inappropriate nursing diagnosis and outcome criteria.
- Lack of regard or respect for the patient.

INTERPERSONAL COMMUNICATION

- Interpersonal communication is a transaction between the sender and the receiver. Both persons participate simultaneously.
- In the transactional model, both participants perceive each other, listen to each other, and simultaneously engage in the process of creating meaning in

a relationship, focusing on the patients issues and assisting them learn new coping skills.
- Both sender and receiver bring certain preexisting conditions to the exchange that influence the intended message and the way in which message is interpreted.

Context of Therapeutic Communication

Values, attitudes and beliefs
- *Example*: Attitudes of prejudice are expressed through negative stereotyping.

Culture or religion
- Cultural mores, norms, ideas, and customs provide the basis for ways of thinking.

Social status
- High-status persons often convey their high-power position with gestures of hands on hips, power dressing, greater height, and more distance when communicating with individuals considered to be of lower social status.

Gender
- Masculine and feminine gestures influence messages conveyed in communication with others.

Age or developmental level
- *Example:* The influence of developmental level on communication is especially evident during adolescence, with words such as "cool", "awesome," and others.

The environment
- Territoriality, density, and distance are aspects of environment that communicate messages.
  - *Territoriality*—the innate tendency to own space
  - *Density*—the number of people within a given environmental space
  - *Distance*—the means by which various cultures use space to communicate

Proxemics: Use of space
- *Intimate distance*—the closest distance that individuals allow between themselves and other.
- *Personal distance*—the distance for interactions that are personal in nature, such as close conversation with friends.
- *Social distance*—the distance for conversation with strangers or acquaintances.
- *Public distance*—the distance for speaking in public or yelling to someone some distance away.

Nonverbal Communication: Body language
Components of nonverbal communication :
- Physical appearance and dress
- Body movement and posture
- Touch
- Facial expressions
- Eye behavior
- Vocal cues or paralanguage.

Therapeutic Communication and Problem-Solving

Goals are often achieved through use of the *problem-solving model:*
- Identify the client's problem.
- Promote discussion of desired changes.
- Discuss aspects that cannot realistically be changed and ways to cope with them more adaptively.
- Discuss alternative strategies for creating changes the client desires to make.
- Weigh benefits and consequences of each alternative.
- Help client select an alternative.
- Encourage client to implement the change.
- Provide positive feedback for client's attempts to create change.
- Help client evaluate outcomes of the change and make modifications as required.

Listening to the Patient

To listen actively is to be attentive to what client is saying, both verbally and nonverbally.

Several nonverbal behaviors have been designed to facilitate attentive listening.
- S – Sit squarely facing the client.
- O – Observe an open posture.
- L – Lean forward toward the client.
- E – Establish eye contact.
- R – Relax.

Process Recordings
- Written reports of verbal interactions with clients
- A means for the nurse to analyze the content and pattern of interaction
- A learning tool for professional development
- How do I give a patient feedback.

Feedback is useful when it is
- Descriptive rather than evaluative and focused on the behavior rather than on the client
- Specific rather than general
- Directed toward behavior that the client has the capacity to modify imparts information rather than offers advice.

Nontherapeutic Communication Techniques
- **Giving reassurance**—may discourage client from further expression of feelings if client believes the feelings will only be downplayed or ridiculed.
- **Rejecting**—refusing to consider client's ideas or behavior.
- **Approving or disapproving**—implies that the nurse has the right to pass judgment on the "goodness" or "badness" of client's behavior.

- **Agreeing or disagreeing**—implies that the nurse has the right to pass judgment on whether client's ideas or opinions are "right" or "wrong".
- **Giving advice**—implies that the nurse knows what is best for client and that client is incapable of any self-direction.
- **Probing**—pushing for answers to issues the client does not wish to discuss causes client to feel used and valued only for what is shared with the nurse.
- **Defending**—to defend what client has criticized implies that client has no right to express ideas, opinions, or feelings.
- **Requesting an explanation**—asking "why" implies that client must defend his or her behavior or feelings.
- **Indicating the existence of an external source of power**—encourages client to project blame for his or her thoughts or behaviors on others.
- **Belittling feelings expressed**—causes client to feel insignificant or unimportant.
- **Making stereotyped comments, clichés, and trite expressions**—these are meaningless in a nurse-client relationship.
- **Using denial**—blocks discussion with client and avoids helping client identify and explore areas of difficulty.
- **Interpreting**—results in the therapist's telling client the meaning of his or her experience.
- **Introducing an unrelated topic**—causes the nurse to take over the direction of the discussion.

Therapeutic Communication Techniques

Communication is the most powerful tool a psychiatric nurse should have. It is the basis of therapeutic–nurse patient relationship. Communication is a complex process and needs practice to use it effectively. Therapeutic communication techniques are methods used to encourage patients to interact in a manner that promotes their growth and moves them toward their treatment goals. All the communication must be aimed at preserving the self-respect of both the helper and helpee.

Listening

Listening is an active process of receiving information and examining reaction to the messages received. It is not simply hearing. It is essential to reach any understanding of the patient. It is the first rule of therapeutic-nurse relationship. The patient should be talking more than the nurse during the interaction. Listening is sign of respect and is powerful reinforcer. Active listening involves all the nurse's senses. For example, maintaining eye contact and receptive nonverbal communication which helps to convey the nurse's interest and acceptance.

Broad Opening

Here, the nurse is encouraging the patient to select topics for discussion. Patient should be welcomed to the communication with warmth and respect.

Patient should feel that nurse is ready to listen. Open-ended questions result in fuller, more revealing answers.

For example:
> What are you thinking about?
> Can you tell me more about that?
> What shall we discuss today?

Domination of the interaction by the nurse or rejecting the responses by the nurse results in poor therapeutic relationship.

Questioning

The nurse skillfully asks open-ended questions during the initial admission. Interviewing skills are necessary to avoid asking too many personal questions in one session. Questions should be to achieve relevance and depth.

> How come you stopped taking your medication?
> Tell me how you feel now?

Restating

Nurse is repeating of the main thought the patient has expressed. It also indicates that the nurse is listening, validating, reinforcing or calling attention to what has been said. Usually a part of patient's statement is repeated. When restating patient should not feel the nurse is reassuring, judgmental or defending.

> E.g. "Your mother left you when you were 5-year-old?

Clarification

Here, the nurse makes specific questions to help clear up a specific point patient makes by attempting to put in to words vague ideas or unclear ideas of the patient. Patient's verbalizations may not be clear when overwhelmed with emotions. Nothing should be allowed to pass to the patient that nurse does not hear or understand.

"I am not sure what you mean. Could do tell me about it again?"

Failure to probe and assumed understanding result in poor communication.

Reflection

By reflection nurse is directing back the patient's ideas, feeling, questions or content. Reflection lets the patient know that the nurse has heard what was said and understand the content. Reflection of the feelings let the patient know that the nurse is aware of what the patient is feeling. It signifies understanding, empathy, interest and respect for the patient. Other techniques may not represent empathetic understanding.

> **" You are looking sad and tense. Is it related to what you have explained?"**

Reflecting techniques can be used incorrectly, when stereotyping patient's response, inappropriate timing of reflections and inappropriate cultural experience and educational level of the patient.

Focusing

Focusing helps the patient expand a topic of importance and also helps in analyzing in detail. It helps the patient talk about life experiences or problem areas and accepts the responsibility for improving them. If the goal is to change thoughts, feelings or beliefs, the patient must first identify and down them. It allows the patient discuss central issues and keeps the communication goal-directed.

" I think you should talk more about your relationship with your husband?"

Sharing Perceptions

It involves asking the patient to verify the nurse's understanding of what the patient is thinking or feeling. For example, nurse is interviewing an alcoholic patient:

Patient: My wife and children are so good. They love me. But I do not know what happened to me. I can not care them. I can not stop drinking.

Nurse: You seem to be very disappointed with your drinking. Am I right about that?

If used inappropriately sharing perceptions can make the patient feel challenging, reassuring, testing.

Theme Idenification

Themes are underlying issues or problems experienced by the patient that emerge repeatedly during the course of the nurse-patient relationship, like anxiety, depression.

"It sounds like that is very important to you. You have mentioned it a very few times."

Silence

Here, the nurse use lack of verbal communication for a therapeutic reason. It allows the patient to think and gain insights. Silence on the part of nurse has varying effects, depending on how the patient perceives it. To a vocal patient silence on the part of nurse may be welcome, but with a depressed or withdrawn patient, the nurse's silence may convey support, understanding, and acceptance.

Humor

Humor is basic part of our personality and has a place in therapeutic nurse-patient relationship. It is the discharge of energy through the comic enjoyment of imperfect. It may be helpful with a patient experiencing mild to moderate anxiety. Humor should be consistent with social and cultural values.

Informing

Informing or giving information is nurse shares simple facts with the patient. This skill is use in patient education like when to take medication, necessary precautions and side effects.

"I think you need to know more about your medication works"

Informing should not fall in to giving advice.

Suggesting

Suggesting is the presentation of alternate ideas. As a therapeutic technique, it is useful intervention in the working phase of the relationship. Suggesting or giving advice can be non-therapeutic. Patient may take nurse's advice and still have an unsuccessful outcome, the patient returns to blame nurse.

Confrontation

Confrontation involves anger and aggression. The therapeutic dimension is assertiveness rather than aggression. Confrontation is an attempt by the nurse to make the patient aware of incongruence in his or her feelings, attitudes, beliefs, and behaviors. It may also help in discovery of ambivalent feelings in the patient. The nurse must be ready to work with the patient through the crisis after confronting the patient. Without this commitment the confrontation lack therapeutic potential and may damage nurse-patient relationship.

Role Playing

Role playing involves acting out a particular situation. It increases patient's insight into human relations can deepen the ability to see the situation from another person's point of view. Role playing can be used for attitude change and to promote self-awareness.

One of the specific ways in which role playing can be used to resolve conflicts and increase self-awareness is through a dialogue that requires the patient to take the part of each person or each side of the problem. If the conflict is internal, the dialogue occurs in the present tense between the conflicting selves until one part of the conflict outweighs the other. If second person is involved, the patient is told to begin the dialogue by expressing wants and resentments about the other person. Then, the patient changes chairs assume the role other person, and responds to what was said. This way patient can express feelings and opinions and gives reality base for the probable response from the other party involved in the conflict.

JOHARI WINDOW

The Johari Window is a communication model that can be used to improve understanding between individuals within a team or in a group setting. Based on disclosure, self-disclosure and feedback, the Johari Window can also be used to improve a group's relationship with other groups.

Developed by Joseph Luft and Harry Ingham (the word "Johari" comes from Joseph Luft and Harry Ingham), there are two key ideas behind the tool:
- That individuals can build trust with others by disclosing information about themselves.
- That they can learn about themselves and come to terms with personal issues with the help of feedback from others.

By explaining the idea of the Johari Window to your team, you can help team members understand the value of self-disclosure, and gently encourage people to give and accept feedback. Done sensitively, this can help people build more-trusting relationships with one another, solve issues and work more effectively as a team.

Explaining the Johari Window

The Johari Window model consists of a foursquare grid (think of taking a piece of paper and dividing it into four parts by drawing one line down the middle of the paper from top to bottom, and another line through the middle of the paper from side-to-side). This is shown in Figure 4.1 below:

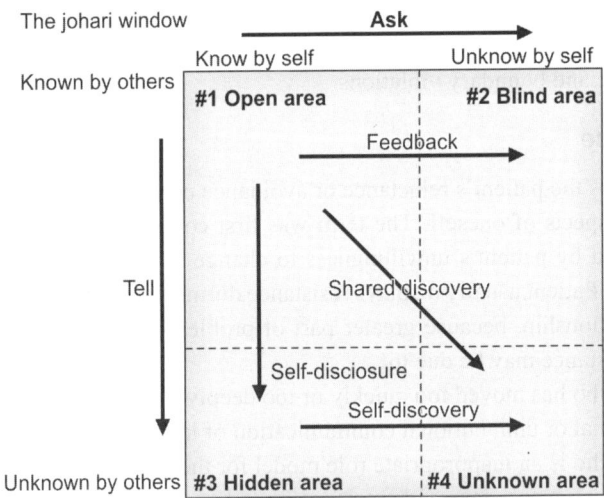

Figure 4.1: Explaining the Johari window

Using the Johari model, each person is represented by their own four-quadrant, or four-pane, window. Each of these contains and represents personal information—feelings, motivation, etc.— about the person, and shows whether the information is known or not known by themselves or other people.

The four quadrants are:

Quadrant 1: Open Area
What is known by the person about him/herself and is also known by others.

Quadrant 2: Blind Area, or Blind Spot
What is unknown by the person about him/herself but which others know. This can be simple information, or can involve deep issues (for example, feelings

of inadequacy, incompetence, unworthiness, rejection) which are difficult for individuals to face directly, and yet can be seen by others.

Quadrant 3: Hidden or Avoided Area
What the person knows about him/herself that others do not.

Quadrant 4: Unknown Area
What is unknown by the person about him/herself and is also unknown by others. The process of enlarging the open quadrant vertically is called self-disclosure, a give and take process between the person and the people he/she interacts with.

THERAPEUTIC IMPASSES

For variety of reasons therapeutic communication can be hindered. Therapeutic impasses are blocks in the progress of nurse-patient relationship. They arise for variety of reasons, but the all crates stall in the process of nurse-patient relationship. Impasse provokes variety of emotions in both the patient and nurse ranging from anxiety and apprehension to frustration, love, or intense anger. The commonest four impasses are discussed here: resistance, transference, counter transference and boundary violations.

Resistance

Resistance is the patient's reluctance or avoidance of verbalizing or experiencing troubling aspects of oneself. The term was first coined by Freud. Resistance is often caused by patient's unwillingness to change when the need for change is recognized. Patient usually displays resistance during the working phase of nurse-patient relationship, because greater part of problem-solving occurs during this phase. Resistance may be due to:
- Nurse who has moved too quickly or too deeply into the patient's feelings.
- Intentional or unintentional communication of lack of respect.
- Nurse who is an inappropriate role model for therapeutic behavior.
- Secondary gain—favorable environmental, interpersonal, and situational changes occur and material advantages as a result of the illness (secondary gain can become a powerful force in perpetuating an illness because it makes environment more comfortable).

Transference

Transference is an unconscious response in which the patient experiences feelings and attitudes toward the nurse that were originally associated with other significant figures in his or her life.
- They may be triggered by superficial similarity, such as facial features or speech, or by personality style or trait.
- These reactions are the patient's attempt to reduce anxiety.

- The nurse may be viewed as an authority figure from the past such as parent figure, or lost loved object, such as former spouse.
- Transference reactions are harmful to the therapeutic relationship only if they are ignored and unexplained.
- Two types of transference are particularly problematic in nurse-patient relationship: hostile transference and dependent reaction transference.

Hostile Transference

Patient may express hostility by uncooperativeness, negativism and hostile silence. If the hostility and anger are internalized, this resistance is expressed as depression and discouragement. Patient may terminate the relationship on the grounds that there is no chance of getting well. If hostility is externalized, the patient may become critical, defiant, and irritable and may express doubts about nurse's training, experience or competence. Patient may attempt to compete with the nurse by reading books on psychology and debating intellectual issues rather than working on real life problems.

Dependent Reaction Transference

This resistance is characterized by patient who are submissive, subordinate, and irritating and who regard nurse as godlike figure. Patient continues to demand more of the nurse.

Management of Transference and Resistance
- Resistance and transference can be difficult problems for the nurse. The psychiatric nurse must be ready to be exposed to such powerful positive and negative emotional responses from the patient.
- Resistance may be due to the nurse and patient have not arrived a mutually acceptable goals or plans of action. The appropriate action here is to return to the goals, purposes and roles of the nurse and patient relationship.
- The analysis of the resistance or transference should be directed toward the patient gaining awareness of these motivations and learning about being completely responsible for all actions or behavior.
- The first thing nurse must listen to the patient.
- When transference or resistance is recognized clarification and reflection of feelings can be used. Clarification gives the nurse a more focussed idea of what is happening. Reflection of the content may help patients become aware of what has been going on their own mind.

For example, nurse may say "I sense you are struggling with yourself. Part of you want to explore the issue of your marriage and another part says 'No I am not ready yet' ".

Countertransference

It is a therapeutic impasse created by the nurse's specific emotional response to the qualities of the patient. This is inappropriate to the content and context of

therapeutic nurse-patient relationship. It is transference applied to the nurse. It is natural that nurse feels warmth toward or liking for some patients more than others. The nurse also will be genuinely angry about the actions of some patient. But in countertransference, the nurse's responses are not justified by reality. Here nurse identify the patient with individuals from their past, and personal needs interfere with their therapeutic relationship.

Types
1. Reactions of intense love or caring
2. Reactions of intense disgust or hostility
3. Reactions of intense anxiety often in response to resistance by the patient.

Examples:
- Difficulty in empathizing with the patient in certain problem areas
- Feeling of depression during or after a session
- Feeling or anger or impatience because of the patient's unwillingness to change
- Argument with the patient or a tendency to push before the patient is ready
- Personal or social involvement with the patient
- Dreams about or preoccupation with the patient
- Sexual or aggressive fantasies about the patient

Other forms include staff involve in countertransfernce
- When they over-react the patient's aggressive behavior, ignore available patient data that would promote understanding
- Ignoring patient's behavior that does not fit the staff's diagnosis, minimizing a patient's behavior, joking about or criticizing a patient or becoming in caught up in intimidation.

The nurse must be constant look out for countertransfernce, become aware when it occurs and work with it to promote therapeutic goals. The nurse must use self-examination throughout the relationship. Following questions are helpful:
- How do I feel about the patient?
- Do I feel sorry or sympathetic for the patient?
- Am I afraid of the patient?
- Do I get extreme pressure out of seeing the patient?
- Do I want to protect, reject, or punish the patient?

Countertransfernce can be harmful to the relationship; it should be dealt as soon as possible. The nurse should discover the source of the problem. When it is recognized the nurse can exercise control over it. If required help, the nurse can seek individual or group supervision.

'Problem patients' may elicit strong negative feelings such as anger, fear and helplessness in the mind of nurse. Such patients should be dealt with patience and action should be directed to making patient responsible for his own behavior. Nurse should review patient's needs and problems and use responsive dimensions of genuineness, respect, empathetic understanding, and concreteness.

Boundary Violations

Here the nurse goes beyond the boundaries of therapeutic relationship and establishes a social, economic, or personal relationship with a patient. Boundary violation is involved whenever a nurse is doing or thinking of doing something special, different or unusual for a patient. Situations where possible boundary violations can happen:
- The patient takes the nurse to a lunch or dinner
- The nurse regularly reveals personal information to the patient
- The nurse accepts free gifts from the patient
- The nurse agrees to meet the patient for treatment outside the usual therapeutic setting without therapeutic justification.

Types
- Role boundaries—problems with role boundaries require the insight of the nurse and the setting of firm therapeutic limits with the patient.
- Time boundaries—odd and unusual hours that have no therapeutic necessity.
- Place and space boundaries—usually in an office or a hospital unit, outside that requires strong therapeutic rationale.
- Money boundaries—regarding fee.
- Gift and service boundaries—gift acceptance may place undue obligations to the patient.
- Clothing boundaries—dress appropriately in a therapeutic manner.
- Language boundaries—addressing the patient and nurse's choice of words in implementing care. Too familiar, sexual, off-color or leading language are boundary violations.
- Self-disclosure boundaries—inappropriately timed self-disclosure and that lacking therapeutic value.
- Post-discharge social boundaries—post-discharge social contact raise the question of boundary violation.
- Physical contact boundaries—sexual contact.

Chapter 5

Psychotic Disorders

Psychosis refers to a loss of contact with reality. When people can not tell the difference between what is real and what is not, it is called a psychotic episode. A first episode of psychosis is often very frightening, confusing and distressing, particularly because it is an unfamiliar experience.

Psychosis usually first appears in a person's late teens or early 20s. Approximately three out of every 100 people will have a psychotic episode in their lifetime. Psychosis occurs in men and women and across all cultures and socioeconomic groups.

FUNCTIONAL PSYCHOSIS OR SCHIZOPHRENIA

Schizophrenia is a group of severe brain disorders in which people interpret reality abnormally. Schizophrenia may result in some combination of hallucinations, delusions and disordered thinking and behavior. The ability of people with schizophrenia to function normally and to care for themselves tends to deteriorate over time.

Contrary to some popular belief, schizophrenia is not split personality or multiple personality. The word "schizophrenia" does mean "split mind", but it refers to a disruption of the usual balance of emotions and thinking. Some selected facts regarding schizophrenia are given in Table 5.1 and common misconceptions regarding schizophrenia are given in Table 5.2.

Risk Factors

Although the precise cause of schizophrenia is not known, researchers have identified certain factors that seem to increase the risk of developing or triggering schizophrenia, including:

Table 5.1: Some facts about schizophrenia

- Schizophrenia is diagnosed in people aged 17–35 years
- The illness appears earlier in men than in women
- Many of the affected people are disabled
- Schizophrenics may not be able to hold down jobs or even perform tasks as simple as conversations
- Many are homeless
- Some schizophrenics recover enough to live a life free from assistance
- People with schizophrenia may not make sense when they talk
- Sometimes people with schizophrenia seem perfectly fine until they talk
- People with schizophrenia are not usually violent.

Table 5.2: Common misconceptions about schizophrenia
MYTH: Schizophrenia refers to a "split personality" or multiple personalities.
FACT: Multiple personality disorder is a different and much less common disorder than schizophrenia. People with schizophrenia do not have split personalities. Rather, they are "split off" from reality.
MYTH: Schizophrenia is a rare condition.
FACT: Schizophrenia is not rare; the lifetime risk of developing schizophrenia is widely accepted to be around 1 in 100.
MYTH: People with schizophrenia are dangerous.
FACT: Although the delusional thoughts and hallucinations of schizophrenia sometimes lead to violent behavior, most people with schizophrenia are neither violent nor a danger to others.
MYTH: People with schizophrenia cannot be helped.
FACT: While long-term treatment may be required, the outlook for schizophrenia is not hopeless. When treated properly, many people with schizophrenia are able to enjoy life and function within their families and communities.

- Having a family history of schizophrenia
- Exposure to viruses, toxins or malnutrition while in the womb, particularly in the first and second trimesters
- Stressful life circumstances
- Older paternal age
- Taking psychoactive drugs during adolescence and young adulthood.

Etiology: Theories About Schizophrenia

Biological
Biological theories of schizophrenia focus on genetic factors, neuroanatomic, neurochemical factors and immunovirology.
- **Genetic contribution:**
  - Genetic studies have concentrated on immediate families—parents, siblings, offsprings.
  - Twin studies: Identical twins have a 50% risk of schizophrenia (even though their genes are 100% equal) than Fraternal twins or other sibs with 15% risk.
  - Adoption studies.
  - May be *polygenic.*
- **Neurochemical and Neuroanatomic factors**
  Alterations in neurotransmitter systems of the brains of people with schizophrenia. Currently the most prominent neurochemical theories involve dopamine and serotonin.
  Dopamine (DA) Hypothesis:
  All can also lead to psychotic behaviors
  - Too much DA linked to schizophrenic symptoms
  - Neurons using DA fire too often

- Transmit too many messages, confusing the brain
- Produces symptoms of disorder
- Substance that decrease DA levels decrease symptoms of schizophrenia.
- Reserpine affects vesicles–reduces schizophrenia
- Substance that block access to DA receptors effective in schizophrenia
- High correlation between blocking and effective treatment.
- agonist of DA (apomorphine) or that increase DA formation (L-Dopa), or increase release (amphetamine), or block DA (cocaine) worsen schizophrenia
- May best explain Type I
- Type II does not seem to be related to abnormal DA chemistry in the brain.

Serotonin Hypothesis
- Serotonin modulates and help to control excess dopamine
- Some believes excess serotonin contributes to schizophrenia.

Structural Abnormalities-neuroanatomic
- Many Type II patients have structural abnormalities in brain:
- Enlarged ventricles (site in brain where cerebrospinal fluid (CSF) is produced)
- Found that people with schizophrenia has less brain tissue and CSF
- PET studies suggest diminished glucose metabolism and oxygen in frontal cortical areas of the brain
- Research shows decreased brain volume and abnormal brain function in the frontal and temporal areas of the brain of persons with schizophrenia
- May be related to prenatal brain development or brain damage
- Also linked to abnormal blood flow within brain, smaller temporal and frontal lobes, and less gray matter.

- **Viral Infection**
  - May result from prenatal exposure to certain viruses (do not know which for sure) that come out of dormancy in teens, adulthood
  - Mothers of schizophrenic patients report more instances of flu during winter
  - Increased levels of antibodies to certain viruses found in blood of schizophrenic patients
  - Not specific to Type I or Type II.
- **Psychological Theories**
  - **Stress**—increased number of stressful life events probably triggering effect on onset of schizophrenia in predisposed individual.
  - Increased Expressed Emotions (EE) (hostility, critical comments, emotional over involvement of "significant others".
  - **Family theories**: "Schizophrenogenic mothers", lack of "real parents", dependency on mother, anxious mother, parental marital discord are examples.
  - **Information processing hypothesis**—disturbances in attention, inability to maintain a set, and inability to assimilate and integrate percepts are common finding in schizophrenia.

- There is possibility of breakdown in the internal representation of mental events.
- **Psychoanalytical theories**—according to Freud, there is regression to the pre-oral (and oral) stage of psychosexual development with the use of defense mechanisms of denial, reaction formation, and projection.
- **Sociocultural**
  - Social influences (like poverty, abuse, family problems) affect an individual's mental functioning.
  - Not much evidence to support it as a cause, but it definitely affects the course of the disease.
  - May have a diathesis-stress explanation: Biological predisposition and psychological/sociocultural stresses.

Course of Schizophrenia

Usually 3 phases:
- Prodromal—no obvious symptoms, but everyday functioning is beginning to deteriorate
- Active—full-blown schizophrenia, with active symptoms
- Residual—symptoms subside, prodromal-like state.

Symptoms can return—back into active phase.

Subtypes of Schizophrenia

These can be either Type I or II depending on what symptoms manifest
- **Paranoid Schizophrenia:**
  - Hallucinations-persecutory content, grandiose content
  - Delusions-persecution, reference, grandiosity, control, infidelity, well-systemized
  - Disturbances of affect, volition, speech, and motor behavior
  - Tends to be organized in thought, speech, just bizarre
  - Usually Type I
  - John Nash (A Beautiful Mind) had this type.
- **Catatonic Schizophrenia:**
  - Psychomotor disturbance is prime symptom
  - Usually Type II.
- **Disorganized Schizophrenia:**
  - Flat/Inappropriate Affect
  - Disorganized Thoughts/Speech
  - Confused, Incoherent
  - Prognosis usually poor.
- **Undifferentiated Schizophrenia:**
  - Not easily classified into other types;
  - Mix of symptoms.
- **Residual Schizophrenia:**
  - Maps onto residual phase of disorder
  - Symptoms decrease in intensity and number

- Some trace remains
- Can be residual while on medication.
- **Post Schizophrenia Depression.**

Signs and Symptoms

Bleuler classification of symptoms (Bleuler 1911)	
Fundamental symptoms	Accessory symptoms
Include 4 **a's**—disturbances of **as**sociations, changes in emotional (**a**ffective) reactions, **a**utism (withdrawal from reality), and **a**mbivalence	Hallucinations, delusions, catatonia and abnormal behaviors

Schneider (1887–1967)
Schneider's first rank symptoms of schizophrenia
Thought echo- hearing thoughts spoken aloud
Third person auditory hallucinations
Hallucinations in the form of a commentary
Somatic hallucinations
Thought withdrawal or insertion
Thought broadcasting
Delusional perception
Feelings or actions experienced a made or influenced by external agents-soamatic passivity

Disorders of thought and verbal behavior—usually identified from speech and writing.

Delusions—false beliefs, unshakable, not affected by rational argument or evidence, firmly held on inadequate grounds that may accompany psychotic disorders:
- *Primary, secondary and shared* delusions
- Grandeur—great/special person
- Reference—special/personal meanings
- Control—controlled by others
- Bizarre—unusual.

Steam of thought—perseveration, loosening of associations, derailment, word salad, neologisms.

Disorders of perception
- Hallucinations-perception in the absence of stimuli to the sense organs in a similar quality to a true percept.
  - Auditory—second person, third person may hear voices, respond and act on voices
  - Visual—false sensory experiences such as seeing something without any external visual stimulus

- Olfactory
- Somatic —tactile and deep
- Pseudohallucinations
- Illusions—misperceptions of external stimuli.

Disorders of affect
- Congruence, apathy, blunted or flattened
- Avolition—loss of motivation, "drained"
- Flat affect—separation from external world.

Disorders of motor behavior—psychomotor:
Psychomotor agitation or retardation
- Agitation—purposeless or disorganized movement
- Retardation—slowed or lack of movement
- In extreme form—catatonia
- Catatonic stupor—stopped responding to environmental stimulus
- Waxy flexibility—posed like a wax statue
- Rigidity—do not move
- Posturing—assume bizarre postures for long periods of time.

Positive and Negative Symptoms
Positive symptoms: In schizophrenia, positive symptoms reflect an excess or distortion of normal functions. These active, abnormal symptoms may include:
- **Delusions:** These beliefs are not based in reality and usually involve misinterpretation of perception or experience. They are the most common of schizophrenic symptoms.
- **Hallucinations**: These usually involve seeing or hearing things that do not exist, although hallucinations can be in any of the senses. Hearing voices is the most common hallucination among people with schizophrenia.
- **Thought disorder:** Difficulty speaking and organizing thoughts may result in stopping speech midsentence or putting together meaningless words, sometimes known as "word salad".
- **Disorganized behavior:** This may show in a number of ways, ranging from childlike silliness to unpredictable agitation.

Negative symptoms: Negative symptoms refer to a diminishment or absence of characteristics of normal function. They may appear months or years before positive symptoms. They include:
- Loss of interest in everyday activities
- Appearing to lack emotion
- Reduced ability to plan or carry out activities
- Neglect of personal hygiene
- Social withdrawal
- Loss of motivation.

Cognitive symptoms: Cognitive symptoms involve problems with thought processes. These symptoms may be the most disabling in schizophrenia, because they interfere with the ability to perform routine daily tasks. A person with

schizophrenia may be born with these symptoms, but they may worsen when the disorder starts. They include:
- Problems with making sense of information
- Difficulty paying attention
- Memory problems.

Medications

Medications are the cornerstone of schizophrenia treatment. But because medications for schizophrenia can cause serious but rare side effects, people with schizophrenia may be reluctant to take them.

Antipsychotic medications are the most commonly prescribed to treat schizophrenia. They are thought to control symptoms by affecting the brain neurotransmitters dopamine and serotonin. A person's willingness to cooperate with treatment may affect medication choice. Someone who is uncooperative may need to be given injections instead of taking a pill. Someone who is agitated may need to be calmed initially with benzodiazapine such as lorazepam (Ativan), which may be combined with an antipsychotic.

Atypical Antipsychotics

These newer medications are generally preferred, because they pose a lower risk of debilitating side effects than do conventional medications. They include: Aripiprazole (Abilify), Clozapine (Clozaril), Olanzapine (Zyprexa), Paliperidone (Invega), Quetiapine (Seroquel), Risperidone (Risperdal), Ziprasidone (Geodon).
Side effects of atypical antipsychotic medications include weight gain, diabetes and high blood cholesterol.

Conventional, or Typical, Antipsychotics

These medications have frequent and potentially significant neurological side effects, including the possibility of developing a movement disorder (tardive dyskinesia) that may or may not be reversible. This group of medications includes: Chlorpromazine (Thorazine), Fluphenazine, Haloperidol, Perphenazine.

These typical antipsychotics are often cheaper than newer counterparts, especially the generic versions, which can be an important consideration when long-term treatment is necessary.

It can take several weeks after first starting a medication to notice an improvement in symptoms. In general, the goal of treatment with antipsychotic medications is to effectively control signs and symptoms at the lowest possible dosage. The psychiatrist may try different medications, different dosages or combinations over time to achieve the desired result. Other medications also may be helpful, such as antidepressants or anti-anxiety medications.

Psychosocial treatments: Although medications are the cornerstone of schizophrenia treatment, once psychosis recedes, psychosocial treatments also are important. These may include:

- **Social skills training:** This focuses on improving communication and social interactions.
- **Family therapy:** This provides support and education to families dealing with schizophrenia.
- **Vocational rehabilitation and supported employment:** This focuses on helping people with schizophrenia find and keep jobs.
- **Individual therapy:** Learning to cope with stress and identify early warning signs of relapse can help people with schizophrenia manage their illness.

MOOD DISORDERS

Mood disorders refer to a category of mental health problems that include all types of depression and bipolar disorder. Mood disorders are sometimes called affective disorders.

Causes of Mood Disorders

Although there is no concrete evidence to nail the cause of mood disorders, genetics, imbalance in brains chemicals (neurotransmitters), hormonal imbalances and the environment in which an individual lives can be causative factors of the problem.

Manic episode: A manic episode is characterized by period of time where an elevated, expansive or notably irritable mood is present, lasting for at least one week. These feelings must be sufficiently severe to cause difficulty or impairment in occupational, social, educational or other important functioning and can not be better explained by a mixed episode. Symptoms also can not be the result of substance use or abuse (e.g. alcohol, drugs, medications) or caused by a general medical condition. Three or more of the following symptoms must be present:
- Elevated, expansive or irritable mood
  There are 4 stages depending on the severity of manic episode
    - Euphoria (mild elevation of mood) stage I: Increased sense of psychological well being and happiness not in keeping with ongoing events.
    - Elation (moderate elevation of mood) Stage II: Feeling of confidence and enjoyment along with increased psychomotor activity.
    - Exaltation (severe elevation of mood) stage III: Intense elation with delusions of grandeur
    - Ecstasy (very severe elevation of mood) stage IV: Intense sense rapture.

There may be rapid, short lasting shifts from euphoria to depression or anger.
- Inflated self-esteem or grandiosity
- Decreased need for sleep (e.g. one feels rested after only 3 hours of sleep)
- More talkative than usual or pressure to keep talking
- Flight of ideas or subjective experience that thoughts are racing
- Attention is easily drawn to unimportant or irrelevant items

- Increase in goal-directed activity (either socially, at work or school, or sexually) or psychomotor agitation
- Excessive involvement in pleasurable activities that have a high potential for painful consequences (e.g. engaging in unrestrained buying sprees, sexual indiscretions, or foolish business investments).

Depressive episode: A person who suffers from a depressive episode must either have a depressed mood or a loss of interest or pleasure in daily activities consistently for at **least a 2 week period**. This mood must represent a change from the person's normal mood; social, occupational, educational or other important functioning must also be negatively impaired by the change in mood. A major depressive episode is also characterized by the presence of 5 or more of these symptoms:

- Depressed mood most of the day, nearly every day, as indicated by either subjective report (e.g. feeling sad or empty) or observation made by others (e.g. appears tearful). (In children and adolescents, this may be characterized as an irritable mood)
- Markedly diminished interest or pleasure in all, or almost all, activities most of the day, nearly every day
- Significant weight loss when not dieting or weight gain (e.g. a change of more than 5% of body weight in a month), or decrease or increase in appetite nearly everyday
- Insomnia (inability to sleep) or hypersomnia (sleeping too much) nearly everyday
- Psychomotor agitation or retardation nearly everyday
- Fatigue or loss of energy nearly everyday
- Feelings of worthlessness or excessive or inappropriate guilt nearly everyday
- Diminished ability to think or concentrate, or indecisiveness, nearly everyday
- Recurrent thoughts of death (not just fear of dying), recurrent suicidal ideation without a specific plan, or a suicide attempt or a specific plan for committing suicide.

OTHER TYPES OF MOOD DISORDERS

Depressive Disorders

Major Depressive Disorder

This disorder is characterized by depressed mood or loss of interest or pleasure in usual activities. Evidence will show impaired social and occupational functioning that has existed for at least two weeks, no history of manic behavior, and symptoms that cannot be attributed to use of substances or a general medical condition.

Major Depressive Disorder may be further classified as follows:

1. Single episodic or recurrent: A single episode specifier is used for an individual's first diagnosis of depression. Recurrent is specified when the history reveals two or more episodes of depression.
2. Mild, moderate or severe: These categories are identified by the number and severity of symptoms.
3. With psychotic features: The impairment of reality testing is evident. The individual experiences delusions or hallucinations.
4. With catatonic features: This category identifies the presence of psychomotor disturbances such as severe psychomotor retardation, with or without the presence of waxy flexibility or stupor or excessive motor activity. The individual may also manifest symptoms of negativism, mutism, echolalia or echopraxia.
5. With melancholic features: This is a typically severe form of major depressive episode. Symptoms are exaggerated. Even temporary reactivity to usually pleasurable stimuli is absent. History reveals a good respose to antidepressant or other somatic therapy.
6. Chronic: This classification applies when the current episode of depressed mood has been evident continuously for at least the past 2 years.
7. With seasonal patterns: This diagnosis indicates the presence of depressive symptoms during the fall or winter month. This diagnosis is made when the number of seasonal depressive episode is substantially higher than the number of nonseasonal depressive episodes that have occurred over the individuals lifetime.
8. With postpartum onset: This specifier is used when symptoms of major depression occur within 4 weeks of postpartum.

Dysthymic Disorder

Individuals with dysthymic disorder describe the mood as sad or "down in the dumps". There is no evidence of psychotic symptoms. The essential feature is a chronically depressed mood for most of the day, more days than not for at least 2 years. It is classified into:

1. **Early onset:** Identifies cases of dysthymic disorder when the onset occurs before age 21 years.
2. **Late onset:** Identifies cases of dysthymic disorder when the onset occurs at age 21 years or older.

Premenstrual Dysphoric Disorder

The DSM IV TR does not include premenstrual dysphoric disorder as an official diagnostic category, but provides a set of research criteria to promote further study of the disorder. The essential feature include markedly depressed mood, marked anxiety, mood swings and decreased interest in activities during the week prior to menses and subsiding shortly after the onset of menstruation.

Bipolar Disorders

The bipolar disorder is characterized by mood swings from profound depression to extreme euphoria with intervening periods of normalcy. Delusions or hallucinations may or may not be part of the clinical picture and onset of symptoms may reflect a seasonal pattern.

Bipolar I Disorder

It is diagnosis given to an individual who is experiencing or has experienced, a full syndrome of manic and mixed symptoms. The client also may have experienced episodes of depression.

Bipolar II Disorders

This diagnostic category is characterized by recurrent bouts of major depression with episodic occurrence of hypomania. The client has never experienced an episode that meets the full criteria for mania or mixed symptomatology.

Cyclothymic Disorder

The essential feature of cyclothymic disorder is a chronic mood disturbance of at least 2 years duration involving numerous episodes of hypomania and depressed mood of insufficient severity or duration to meet the criteria for either bipolar I or II disorder.

Other Mood Disorders

Mood Disorders due to a General Medical Condition

This disorder is characterized by a prominent and persistent disturbance in mood that is judged to be the result of direct physiological effects of a general medical condition. The mood disturbance may involve depression or elevated, expansive or irritable mood and causes clinically significant distress or impairment in social, occupational or other important areas of functioning.

Substance-induced Mood Disorders

The disturbance of mood associated with this disorder is considered to be the direct result of physiological effects of a substance. The mood disturbance may involve depression or elevated, expansive or irritable mood and cause clinically significant distress or impairment in social, occupational or other areas of functioning.

TREATMENT OF BIPOLAR DISORDER

When people with bipolar disorder experience acute mania, immediate referral to a specialist psychiatric service is usually necessary. Diagnosing bipolar disorder can be very complex and the first assessment may not provide a definitive diagnosis. To confirm the diagnosis, a mental health professional (usually a psychiatrist) should undertake a comprehensive assessment.

Hospitalization
- Abnormal Behavior (loss of career, family disintegration)
- Delirious mania.

Comprehensive Clinical Assessment

Their full medical history will be taken which include:
a. A **'risk assessment'**, which assesses a person's potential for experiencing harms associated with mania. These may include aggression, financial harm, risky sexual behavior or vulnerability to exploitation, and the possibility of contracting communicable diseases (such as HIV, Herpes or Hepatitis C) due to sexual behavior.
b. Past episodes of psychiatric problems. If the person has established bipolar disorder, the doctor will also check their compliance with mood stabilizer medications and cease any antidepressants.
c. Physical examination: Its purpose is to exclude organic causes of the manic behavior, such as a neurological disorder, systemic disease, the misuse of alcohol or drugs or other substances, or the use of prescription medication.
d. Also assess any physical consequences of mania (e.g. dehydration, emaciation or injuries).
e. A routine physical investigation (urea and electrolytes, full blood count, liver function tests, thyroid function test, and therapeutic drug monitoring of mood stabilizer serum concentrations).
f. Finally, other investigations will be carried out if needed. These may include a brain scan, cognitive/dementia screen, and an electroencephalography (EEG).

Once this comprehensive assessment is carried out, a treatment plan is developed with the person to tailor the treatment of bipolar disorder to his or her individual needs.

Phases of Treatment

1. **Acute phase:** The goal of the acute phase of treatment is symptom reduction and stabilization. Therefore, for the first few weeks of treatment, mood stabilizers may need to be combined with antipsychotics or benzodiazepines, particularly if the patient has psychotic symptoms, agitation or insomnia. If the clinical situation is not an emergency, it is desirable to start patients on a low dose and gradually increase the dose until the maximum therapeutic benefits has been achieved. Once stabilization is achieved, the frequency of serum level monitoring should be 1 to 2 weeks during the first 2 months and every 3 to 6 months during the long-term maintenance.
2. **Continuum phase:** The goal of this phase is to prevent relapse of the current episode or cycling into the opposite pole. It lasts about 2 to 9 months after acute symptoms have resolved. The usual pharmacologic procedure in this phase is to continue the mood stabilizer while closely monitoring the patient for signs or symptoms of relapse.

3. **Maintenance phase:** The goal of this phase is to sustain remission and to prevent new episodes. It is recommended that long term or life time prophylaxis with a mood stabilizer be instituted after two manic episodes or after one manic episode if it is severe or if there is family history of bipolar disorder.
4. **Discontinuation:** Like major depressive disorder, the course of bipolar disorder is typically recurrent and progressive. Therefore, the same issues and principles regarding the decision to continue or discontinue pharmacotherapy apply.

Somatic Treatment

Acute Treatment of Manic Episodes

Medications are the main way of managing an acute manic episode. The aim of the medications is to stabilize mood.

Components to the drug management of acute mania

- Commencement of a mood stabilizer (lithium, sodium valproate, carbamazepine or olanzapine). Mood stabilizers act upon the elevated mood but take about one week to start working for most people.
- Concurrent use of an antipsychotic or benzodiazepine (or a combination of these). These medications calm or sedate the person with mania as a temporary procedure, until the mood stabilizer starts to help the person to feel better.

Mood stabilizer	Newer anticonvulsants	(With or without) Additional treatments for other symptoms
LITHIUM: Commence with 750–1000 mg daily. Determine serum level after 5 to 7 days of steady-dose treatment [Aim for serum concentration of 0.8–1.2 mmol/L] **Or** **VALPROATE:** Commence with 400–800 mg daily. Determine serum level after 5 days of steady-dose treatment, or use loading dose strategy commencing at 20–30 mg/kg [Aim for serum concentration of 300–800 µmol/L] **Or** **CARBAMAZEPINE** Commence with 200–400 mg daily. Determine serum level after 5 to 7 days of treatment. [Aim for serum concentration of 17–50 µmol/L].	**LAMOTRIGINE (Lamictal)** has been shown to have efficacy in the treatment of mania, both as single agent and in combination with lithium or valproate, particularly effective for rapid cycling and in the depressed phase of bipolar illness. **GABAPENTIN (Neurontin)** has been showed efficacious for acute mania and mood stabilization, including rapid cycling. **TOPIRAMATE (Topamax):** has been used mostly as add—on therapy in mixed patient samples wth refractory mood disorders. A unique characteristic of topiramate is that it is more associated with weight loss than weight gain. **Or** **Olanzapines**—20 mg daily	Treat psychosis Manage sleeping difficulties Oral a. **Benzodiazepines** (diazepam, clonazepam, lorazepam) b. **Antipsychotics** (risperidone, olanzapine, chlorpromazine, thioridazine, haloperidol) **Taken by injection** (only use if oral administration is not possible, or is ineffective) a. **Benzodiazepines** (midazolam IM, diazepam IV) b. **Antipsychotics** (olanzapine IM, haloperidol IM, zuclopenthixol IM)

If the manic episode does not respond to first line treatment
The timing of the decision to change treatment will depend on both clinical urgency and the degree of response, which varies from person to person. It can be
- Increase the dose and/or blood levels of the mood stabilizer
- Add an additional antipsychotic such as risperidone, olanzapine or haloperidol.

If these strategies have being tried and there is still no relief from symptoms, electroconvulsive therapy (ECT) may be considered.
The benzodiazepine or antipsychotic should be withdrawn once the acute episode has resolved and just the mood stabilizer should be continued.

Management of mixed bipolar disorder
Medication options for the treatment of a mixed episode
The treatment of mixed episodes involves the choice of any of these medications:
- Valproate
- Carbamazepine
- Lithium
- Olanzapine

Treatment of Bipolar Depression
Comprehensive clinical assessment - bipolar depressive episode
Clinical assessment requires patient cooperation and may not be possible if the patient is severely slowed physically and mentally.
It is essential to obtain collaborative information especially in cases where cognitive impairment is suspected:
- Suicide risk assessment
- Exclude organic causes (neurological disorder, systemic disease, substance misuse, drug induced)
- Sophisticated appraisal of possible psychotic symptoms—especially pathological/delusional guilt and hallucinations
- Check compliance with mood stabilizers
- Conduct routine hematological and biochemical investigations (urea and electrolytes, full blood count, thyroid function tests, therapeutic drug monitoring)
- Additional investigations if indicated (e.g. brain scan, cognitive/dementia screen).

Pharmacological intervention—depressive episode

New depressive episode	Breakthrough depressive episode on single mood stabilizer	Failure to respond
Initiate and optimize **Mood stabilizer** (lithium, lamotrigine) Or **Mood stabilizer and antidepressant** concurrently (MAOI, TCAS, SSRI)	**Add Antidepressant** [(SSRIs) and venlafaxine form the first-line choice of treatment] MAOIs and TCAS should be considered as second-line treatment choices. Or **Add second mood stabilizer** (After blood levels) For example: Lamotrigine, combining of lithium and carbamazepine	**Switch/substitute antidepressants** Or Switch/substitute Mood stabilizers Or **Electroconvulsive therapy**

Continuing failure to respond
- Confirm correct diagnosis
- Re-evaluate psychological/social factors responsible for maintaining depression
- Consider adjunctive psychological therapies.

Medications for Long-term Treatment of Bipolar Disorder

Long-term treatment is often called the 'maintenance' phase of treatment or 'relapse prevention'. The goal of long-term treatment for bipolar disorder is to maintain a stable mood and to prevent a relapse of mania or a depressive episode.

> Lithium (aim for serum concentration of 0.6–0.8 mmol/L)
> Or
> Valproate (usual dose range 1000–2500 mg; serum concentration 350–700 µmol/L)
> Or
> Carbamazepine (usual dose range 600–1200 mg; serum concentration 17–50 µmol/L)
> Or
> Lamotrigine (usual dose range 50–300 mg; serum concentration not useful)

Psychosocial Treatments

Learning to live with a continuous illness that is episodic is a major issue for people with bipolar disorder and their families.
- As an adjunct to somatic treatment.
- Repeated episodes of mania and depression tend to lead to increased rates of divorce, family breakdown, and unemployment, a break in social networks and education, and financial difficulties

a. **Cognitive behavior therapy:** Therapy aims at correcting the depressive negative conditions, e.g. hopelessness, worthlessness and replacing them by new cognitive ideas and behavioral responses. It is used in mild to moderate depression and can be used along with somatic treatment.

b. **Interpersonal Therapy:** Therapy attempts to recognize and explore interpersonal stressors, role disputes and transitions, social isolation or social skill deficits, which acts as precipitants for depression.

c. **Psychoanalytic Psychotherapy:** Therapy aims at changing the personality itself rather than just ameliorating the symptoms. Their usefulness is uncertain.

d. **Behavior Therapy:** This includes the various short-term modalities like social skill training, problem solving techniques, assertiveness training, self control therapy, activity scheduling and decision making techniques. It is useful in mild cases of depression.

e. **Group Therapy:** Group psychotherapy can be useful in mild cases of depression. It is very useful method of psychoeducation in both recurrent depressive disorder and bipolar disorder.

f. Family and Marital Therapy: The main purpose is to ensure continuity of treatment and to reduce the intrafamilial and interpersonal difficulties and to reduce or modify stressors which may help in a faster and complete recovery.

Complementary (Non-prescribed) Medications

- Herbal remedies and other natural supplements have not been well studied and their effects on bipolar disorder are not fully understood.
- Omega-3 fatty acids (found in fish oil) are being studied to determine their usefulness for long-term treatment of bipolar disorder.
- St John's Wort (hypericum perforatum) is a herb which is being studied in regard to depression, but there is some evidence that it can reduce the effectiveness of some medications, can react with some prescribed antidepressants, or may cause a switch into mania.

ORGANIC MENTAL DISORDERS

Organic brain disorders result from structural pathology, as in dementia, or from disturbed central nervous system (CNS) function, as in fever-induced delirium. They do not include mental and behavioral disorders due to alcohol and misuse of drugs, which are classified separately.

OMD is common in the elderly. It is not a part of the normal aging process, however, OMD is not a separate disease, but is a general term used to describe physical conditions that can cause mental changes.

Disorders associated with OMD include:
- Brain injury caused by trauma
    - Bleeding into the brain (intracerebral hemorrhage)
    - Bleeding into the space around the brain (subarachnoid hemorrhage)
    - Blood clot causing pressure on brain (chronic subdural hematoma)
    - Concussion
- Breathing conditions
    - Low oxygen in the body (hypoxia)
    - High carbon dioxide levels in the body (hypercapnia)
- Cardiovascular disorders
    - Abnormal heart rhythm (arrhythmias)
    - Brain injury due to high blood pressure (hypertensive brain injury)
    - Dementia due to many strokes (multi-infarct dementia)
    - Heart infections (endocarditis, myocarditis)
    - Stroke
    - Transient ischemic attack (TIA)
- Degenerative disorders
    - Creutzfeldt-Jacob disease
    - Diffuse Lewy Body disease
    - Huntington's disease
    - Multiple sclerosis

- Normal pressure hydrocephalus
  - Parkinson's disease
  - Pick's disease
  - Senile dementia, Alzheimer's type
- Dementia due to metabolic causes
- Drug and alcohol-related conditions
  - Alcohol withdrawal state
  - Intoxication, drug abuse, or alcohol use
  - Long-term effects of alcohol, Wernicke-Korsakoff syndrome
  - Withdrawal from drugs (especially sedative-hypnotics and corticosteroids)
- Infections
  - Any sudden onset (acute) or long-term (chronic) infection
  - Blood poisoning (septicemia)
  - Swelling of the brain (encephalitis)
  - Swelling of the lining of the brain and spinal cord (meningitis)
- Other medical disorders
  - Cancer
  - Kidney disease
  - Liver disease
  - Thyroid disease (high or low)
  - Vitamin deficiency (B12 and others)

Other conditions that may be related to organic brain syndrome include:
- Depression
- Neurosis
- Psychosis.

Delirium

Delirium, also termed toxic confusional state and acute organic reaction, is an acute or subacute brain failure in which impairment of attention is accompanied by abnormalities of perception and mood.

It is the most common psychosis seen in the general hospital. About 10 to 20% of surgical and medical inpatients have delirium during their admission.

The degree of impairment classically fluctuates, so that there are intermittent lucid periods. Confusion is usually worse at night, with consequent sleep reversal, so that the patient is asleep in the day and awake all night. During the acute phase, thought and speech are incoherent, memory is impaired and misperceptions occur. Episodic visual hallucinations (or illusions) and persecutory delusions may occur. As a consequence, the patient may be frightened, suspicious, restless and uncooperative.

Dementia

Dementia is an acquired global impairment of intellect, memory and personality, but without impairment of consciousness. There is often an associated deterioration in emotional control, social behavior and motivation.

Classification

Primary or secondary
- Primary dementias as those, such as, Alzheimer's disease, in which the dementia itself is the major signs of some organic brain disease not directed related to any other organic illness. (Devanand and Mayeux 1992)
- Secondary dementias are those caused by or related to another disease or condition, such as HIV disease or a cerebral trauma. There are many causes of dementia.

Epidemiology

- Estimated prevalence of dementia is 1.03% of the population. Facts about dementia are given in Table 5.3.
- Rises to between 16% and 25% for those over 85 ages.
- Approximately 5% of person older, age 65 have severe dementia and 15% have mild dementia. The symptoms of aging and dementia are given in Table 5.4.
- The most common is Alzheimer's disease, which accounts for up to 70% of all cases. Alzheimer's disease is caused by the destruction of certain brain cells leading to the loss of the neurotransmitter acetylcholine.
- Multi-Infract Dementia (MID): MID are second commonest causes of dementia, seen in 10–15% of all cases.
- Hypothyroid Dementia: This is one of the important and reversible causes of dementia. It accounts for less than 1% of dementia. Since clinical diagnosis may be difficult, laboratory tests have to be resorted to for correct diagnosis.

Table 5.3: Facts and tips about dementia

- Dementia is a group of symptoms caused by disorders that affected the brain and loss of mental abilities and most commonly occurs late in life.
- Dementia is characterized the progressive decline in cognitive function due to damage or disease in the body beyond what might be expected from normal aging.
- People have dementia may not be able to think well adequate to do normal activities, for example, getting dressed or eating.
- Memory loss is a common symptom of dementia. Though, memory loss by itself does not mean you have dementia.
- Risk factor of dementia is genetics/family history, smoking and alcohol use, atherosclerosis, cholesterol, plasma homocysteine, diabetes, mild cognitive impairment.
- Generally seen in the older people whose age after 60 and person loss your intellectual and social abilities, healthy brain tissue degenerates, causing a steady decline in memory and mental abilities.
- No one treatment for stop this disease. Though some drugs would be helpful keep symptoms from control for small time.

Table 5.4: Symptoms of normal memory changes and dementia

Typical Aging	Symptoms of Dementia
Complains about memory loss but able to provide detailed examples of forgetfulness	May complain of memory loss only if asked; unable to recall specific instances
Occasionally searches for words	Frequent word-finding pauses, substitutions
May have to pause to remember directions, but does not get lost in familiar places	Gets lost in familiar places and takes excessive time to return home
Remembers recent important events; conversations are not impaired	Notable decline in memory for recent events and ability to converse
Interpersonal social skills are at the same level as they have always been	Loss of interest in social activities; may behave in socially inappropriate ways

- AIDS Dementia Complex: About 50–70% of the patients suffering from AIDS Dementia due to HIV virus. The immune dysfunction associated with HIV disease.

Risk Factors

- Increasing age—by the age of 90, around 1 in 3 people affected
- A family history
- High blood pressure, diabetes, smoking, poor diet and excessive alcohol intake
- Vitamin B12 deficiency.

Stages of Dementia

Early stage (2–4 years)
- Forgetfulness
- Decline interest in environment
- Hesitancy in initiating action
- Poor performance at work.

Middle stage (2–12)
- Progressive memory loss
- Hesitancy in response to questions
- Has difficulty in following simple instructions
- Irritable, anxious, wandering, neglect personal hygiene and social isolation.

Final stage (up to 12)
- Marked loss of weight
- Unable to communicate
- Does not recognize family
- Loss the ability to stand and walk
- Death is usually caused by aspiration pneumonia.

Symptoms

- Memory loss, especially of more recent events. Difficulty finding their way around, especially in new or unfamiliar surroundings poor concentration.

- Problems learning new ideas or skills.
- Psychological problems such as becoming irritable, saying or doing inappropriate.
- Severe mental and physical problems, including loss of speech, immobility, incontinence and frailty.
- Urinary and fecal incontinence may develop in late stage.
- Disorientation in time, place and person develop in last stage.
- Thinking is impaired, the flow of ideas is reduced and the reasoning capacity is also impaired.

Alzheimer's Disease

This is a primary degenerative brain disease of unknown etiology that is insidious in onset, followed by gradual deterioration and death in about 10 years. The onset can be in middle adult life or even earlier, but the incidence is higher in later life. Patients particularly at risk of developing Alzheimer's disease are those who have a family history, who have sustained a head injury, or have Down's syndrome.

Organic Amnestic (Dysmnesic) Syndrome

This is characterized by a marked impairment of memory occurring in clear consciousness and not as part of a delirium or dementia. Long-term memory is less affected than short-term memory. Often the patient is blandly unconcerned and commonly confabulates. One of the most common causes is severe thiamin deficiency secondary to chronic alcohol misuse (Korsakoff's syndrome).

OTHER PSYCHOTIC DISORDERS

Acute Polymorphic Psychotic Disorder with Symptoms of Schizophrenia

This diagnosis is considered not only as the first with schizophrenia manifest, but also in favorable cases of the disease, such as long-term remission and spontaneous output of psychosis, it is advisable each subsequent psychosis attributed to this group, but not to schizophrenia or schizoaffective disorder. In the clinic of acute psychosis in this group there are productive the first rank symptoms characteristic of schizophrenia, but there are no negative emotional-volitional disorders. There is affect of anxiety, expansion and confusion. Motor activity is increased until the excitation.

Diagnosis of acute polymorphic psychotic disorder with symptoms of schizophrenia:
1. Rapid changes in symptoms of delirium, including delusions of control, delusional interpretation and delusional perception, which is characteristic of schizophrenia.
2. Hallucinations, including auditory commenting, contradictory and mutually exclusive, compelling and true pseudohallucinations, somatic hallucinations,

a symptom of the openness of thought, the sound of the own thoughts related to the first-rank symptoms in schizophrenia.
3. Symptoms of emotional distress, fear, anxiety, irritability, confusion.
4. Motor stimulation.
5. The above-mentioned productive symptoms of schizophrenia occur no more than a month.

Treatment of acute polymorphic psychotic disorder with symptoms of schizophrenia

In treatment is necessary to apply detoxication therapy, neuroleptics in the middle, and sometimes in the highest dose. It should always be given supportive treatment prolong or conduct occasional short courses of therapy because of the risk of developing schizophrenia, but also insist on an outpatient observation of patients, at least for one year. Pay attention to periods of sleep disorders, mood disorders (anxiety episodes), suspicion. It is these symptoms that may precede exacerbations, and therefore they are a signal for warning of therapy.

Acute and Transient Psychotic Disorder

Currently, the diagnosis is most common during the first hospitalization. The frequency of diagnosis ranges from 4 to 6 cases per 1000 population per year.

Causes

Acute transient psychotic disorders may be associated with stress, such as loss, a situation of violence, imprisonment, mental pain, overexertion, such as long waiting times, exhausting journey. In this sense, in this group are sharp and partly protracted reactive psychoses. However, they may begin and endogenously determine the internal experiences. In this case, the diagnosis is "cosmetic" to manifest symptoms of schizophrenia or schizoaffective disorder first attack. It is appropriate to put such a diagnosis only for the duration of violations of no more than 3 months.

Symptoms

After an initial short period with symptoms of anxiety, restlessness, insomnia and confusion, there is a sharp sensual delirium with rapid changes in the structure of delusion. Acute psychosis lasts from one to two weeks. Ideas of reference, values of persecution, staging, false recognition of delirium and the twin (Kapgra) occur against the background of the mythological, symbolic interpretation of the environment, in the middle of the action is the patient himself. There are frequent experiences of spiritualization animals, plants, inanimate objects, including some ideas of exposure. Hallucinatory experiences, hearing the true and not persistent and rapidly replace each other pseudohallucinations. Amnesia is absent, although the patient did not immediately tell of his experiences, as it were, gradually remembering it. There is affect of happiness, fear, surprise, confusion and bewilderment, but also sense of "dreamlike" experience.

Psychosis in this group is often associated with stress, so the diagnosis indicates psychosis associated with stress or not. Acute transient psychosis is associated with stress, previously designated as reactive. Conventionally, it is believed that the stressor is considered to be the factor that precedes the psychosis of less than 2 weeks. Nevertheless, it is important clinical criteria and also due to the stressor, which include—the sound of the clinical picture of stress situations such as harassment after the real persecution, and gradual extinction of the sound after the termination of the stressor. In the role of the stressor may be the situation of separation and divorce, economic collapse and loss of social prestige, the news of the disaster or catastrophe.

Acute and Transient Psychotic Disorders Treatment

In treatment is necessary to apply detoxication therapy, neuroleptics in the middle, and sometimes in the highest dose. Typical combinations are a combination of chlorpromazine and haloperidol, haloperidol and triftazin or a combination of a large and antipsychotics tranquilizer. Due to the high risk of re-psychotic, some time after discharge (2–3 weeks), usually in the evening, the patient should receive maintenance doses of neuroleptics.

Schizoaffective Disorder

Schizoaffective disorder is diagnosed when there has been an uninterrupted period of symptoms of schizophrenia which, as noted, may include delusions, hallucinations, disorganization of speech, catatonic behavior and negative symptoms. The patient displays these symptoms along with mood symptoms of a major depressive episode, a manic episode or mixed episode and that during the period of the illness the patient has experienced delusions or hallucinations in the absence of these prominent mood symptoms.

Delusional Disorder

Delusional disorder involves potentially real life situations that are, however, unreal in the life of the patient. Thus, a person may, indeed, be poisoned, famous or followed, but this is not reality for the patient. These patient are not add, eccentric or bizarre as we see in schizophrenia but instead falsely believe that important people are in love with them (erotomanic type) or that they themselves are powerful, knowledgeable, or wealthy (grandiose type), that the person is being malevolently treated (persecutory type), that their sexual partner is unfaithful (jealous type), that they have a physical defect or medical condition (somatic type) or that they have symptoms of two or more of these subtype (mixed type).

Brief Psychotic Disorder (Reactive Psychosis)

It refers to symptoms lasting at least one day, but less than one month, and may include delusions, hallucinations, disorganized speech and either disorganized or catatonic behavior.

It may arise within four weeks of childbirth or caused by marked psychological stressors or can occur in the absence of a stressor.

Shared Psychotic Disorder (Folie A Deux)

In shared psychotic disorder, a delusion or false belief system develops in an individual who is closely involved with another individual who is demonstrably delusional. The second individual's delusion is similar, if not identical, to that of the individual with whom they are involved. They essentially share the same delusional system. This can apply to couples, and it can apply to groups of individuals.

Psychotic Disorders Due to Specific General Condition

It is characterized by hallucination or delusions and can be the result of metabolic, neoplastic, or structural accident of the either the central nervous system, or organ systems which impact the nervous system.

Substance-induced Psychotic Disorder

It can occur with onset during intoxication by the drug or with onset during withdrawal from the drug.

Capgras Syndrome (The Delusion of Doubles)

A syndrome that is closely related to delusional disorders, it is characterized by a delusional conviction that other persons in the environment are not their real selves but are their own doubles.

There are 3 types:

1. Typical capgras syndrome (illusion desosies): Here the person sees a familiar person as a stranger who is imposing as the familiar person.
2. Illusion de fregoli: The person falsely identifies strangers familiar persons.
3. Syndrome or subjective doubles: The person's own self is perceived as being replaced by a double.

   The syndrome is commonly seen in psychotic conditions with delusional symptomatology like, paranoid schizophrenia (most frequently) delusional disorders and organic delusional disorder.

   The treatment is of the underlying disorder.

Management with Psychotic Patient

- Encourage participation in group activities
- Help the patient to focus on his strength than his weakness
- Encourage the patient to work more independently gradually
- Improve and encourage the assertiveness, realize basic human rights
- Develop trusting relationship
- Convey an accepting attitude and enable the patient to express feelings openly

- Allow patient to express anger
- Teach patient the normal stages of grief and the behavior associated with each stage
- Spent time with patient
- Provide positive reinforcement
- Frequently orient to reality
- Use clock and calendars with large numbers that are easy to read
- Keep explanation simple
- Discourage rumination of delusional thinking
- Talk about real people and real events
- Monitor for medication side effect
- Identify the self care deficit and provide assistance as required
- Provide guidance and assistance for independent actions
- Provide a structured schedule of activates that does not change from day to day
- Perform ongoing assessment of clients ability to fulfill nutritional needs, ensure personal safety, follow medication region and communicate need for assistance with activities that he can not accomplish independently
- Involve the family members in the care of the patient.

Chapter 6

Neurotic Disorders

Neurosis is a general term referring to mental distress that, unlike psychosis, does not prevent rational thought or daily functioning. This term, coined by William Cullen in the 18th century, has fallen out of favor along with the psychological school of thought called psychoanalysis, founded by Sigmund Freud.

The DSM no longer lists "neurosis" as a category of mental illness, but disorders associated with the term have included obsessive-compulsive, chronic anxiety, phobias, and pyromania.

While the Greek roots (*neuron,* meaning "nerve," and *-osis,* meaning "disease") implies disorder, neurosis affects most of us in some mild form or other. The problem lies in neurotic thoughts or behaviors that significantly impair, but do not altogether prevent, normal daily living.

ANXIETY

Anxiety is a common emotion in everyone's experience. It is a universal human experience.

Definition

Anxiety is a normal phenomenon which is characterized by a state of apprehension or unease arising out of anticipation of danger.

Fear is an apprehension in response to an external danger while in anxiety the danger is largely unknown.

Etiology

1. Behavioral theory
   Unconditioned inherent response of the organism to painful or dangerous stimuli.
2. Biological theory
   - 2% of general population
     15% of their relatives
     Chemically induced anxiety state.
     Infusion of Na lactate, isoproterenol
     Inhalation of 5% CO_2 (hyperventilation, physical exercise)
   - Alteration of GABA—benzodiazepine receptor
   - Alteration of norepinephrine, 5-HT, dopamine
   - Secondary of some of medical disorder such as hyperthyroidism, hypertension and CAD.

4. Psychological factors
   - Interpersonal factors
   - Anxiety can be arise from problems of interpersonal relationships. In adult, anxiety arises when he cannot meet the norms and values in his cultural group
   - Behavioral factors
   - Anxiety develops from disturbed behavior which interfere with a person's life
   - Cognitive factors
   - Once perception of internal and external stimuli, thoughts (negative automatic thoughts) which all predisposes anxiety disorder.
5. External Factors
   - Stress of work
   - Stress from school
   - Stress in a personal relationship such as marriage or friendships
   - Financial stress
   - Stress from an emotional trauma such as loss of loved one, natural disaster, physical abuse or sexual abuse
   - Stress from a serious medical illness
   - Side effect of medication
   - Lack of oxygen.

Types of Anxiety

1. Generalized anxiety disorder.
2. Panic disorder.

Generalized Anxiety Disorder (GAD)

GAD is characterized by a generalized persistent anxiety of at least six months duration.
It is in an insidious onset.

Clinical Features

- Psychic symptoms:
  - Poor concentration, irritability, inability to relax, insomnia, depersonalization, worry, feeling of being unable to cope
- Physical symptoms
  - Motor tension—body aches, restlessness, fatigue
  - Autonomic arousal—palpitation, dyspnea, tachycardia, dry mouth, frequency of micturition, sweating, dizziness, hyperventilation, diarrhea.

Panic Disorder

Panic disorder is defined as a sudden attack of intense discomfort, fear or terror. The episode is usually sudden onset, lasts for a few minutes and is characterized by very severe anxiety.

Clinical Feature

Psychological symptoms	Physical symptoms
Intense anxiety, fear of dying depersonalization	Increased heart rate, chest pain or discomfort, sweating trembling, dyspnea, GI disorders

Treatment

1. Psychotherapy
   - Establish nurse-patient relationship
   - Supportive psychotherapy
2. Relaxation technique
   - Jacobson's progressive relational technique
   - Yoga, pranayama
   - Meditation
3. Behaviors therapy
   - Hyperventilation control
   - Biofeedback
4. Assertiveness training
   It helps the person take more control over life situation. Techniques help the person negotiate interpersonal situations and foster self-assurance.
5. Drug therapy
   Anxiolytic and antidepressants are usually prescribed. Some of the drugs are benzodiazepines, buspirone and propranalol.
   Buspirone is good choice for long-term management of anxiety disorder.

PHOBIC DISORDER

Phobias are irrational fears of a specific object, situation or activity, often leading to persistence avoidance of the feared object, situation or activity.

The common types of phobias are of three categories:
1. Agoraphobia
2. Specific phobia, and
3. Social phobia—two subtypes, non-generalized type (a fear of public situations such as public speaking or performing on stage) and a generalized type (almost all social interactions are feared).

Agoraphobia

"Agoraphobia is defined as a fear and avoidance of being in places or situations from which escape might be difficult or in which help might not be available in the event of sudden incapacitation".

As a result of such fears, the agoraphobic person avoids travel outside the home or requires accompaniment when away from home.

It is characterized by an irrational fear of being in places away from the familiar setting at home.

It includes fear of open spaces, public places, crowded places, and any other places where there is no escape to a safe place.

A full blown panic attack may occur (agoraphobia with panic disorder) or a few symptoms like dizziness or tachycardia may occur (agoraphobia without panic disorder).

As symptoms worsen, there is a gradual restriction of normal day-to-day activities, and even person confines to home, often depend on a person to go outside(phobic companion).

Social Phobia

"The central feature of social phobia is a persistent, irrational fear of activities or social interactions, characterized by fear of performing activities in the presence of other people or interacting with others."

- Common social phobias involve fears of speaking or eating in public, urinating in public lavatories, writing in front of others, or saying foolish things in social situations.
- Many individuals with social phobia are self-critical and perfectionistic-attempting to conduct themselves according to extreme and exacting standards to avoid the negative evaluation of others that they may perceive as epidemic.
- By leaving anxiety-provoking situations (escape) them entirely (avoidance), individuals with social phobia may reduce or prevent the immediate experience of anxiety, but this relief may also reinforce their belief in their inadequacies.
- Individuals with social phobia experience significant impairment in social, educational, and vocational functioning.
- They may find it difficult to initiate or maintain social or romantic relationships, avoid classes that require public presentations, discontinue their education prematurely, or take jobs below their ability to avoid social or performance demands.
- Often individuals rarely seek treatment.

Specific Phobia

"A condition characterized marked and persistent fear that is excessive or unreasonable and is brought on "by the presence or anticipation of a specific object or situation (e.g. flying, heights, animals, receiving an injection, seeing blood)."

The response may take the form of a situationally bound or predisposed panic attack, and the phobia causes marked distress or interferes with role functioning.

Epidemiology

- Phobias are the most common of all anxiety disorders
- Social phobia is the most common of all phobias
- Lifetime prevalence rates of agoraphobia have been reported from a number of studies

- Social phobia in males—11.1 and in females —15.5 and a total of 13.3.
- Specific phobia occurs in 2.4 to 9.2% of children and adolescents, with usual onset between 5 and 13 years of age
- Women receive diagnoses of specific phobia more often than men
- Onset is often sudden and course usually chronic.

Etiology

Classical Conditioning Theory

This theory holds that phobias are learned through the association of negative experience with an object or situation. Responses of avoidance or escape are learned and serve to decrease the discomfort arising from conditioned stimuli. Repeated negative reinforcement of avoidance behavior maintains the fear and makes it resistant to extinction.

Psychodynamic Theory

Deployment of three specific ego defense mechanisms in phobias.
The first of these is *displacement*, which involves the redirection of anxiety associated with an unconscious source to a conscious substitute that is often intrinsically harmless.

Projection is the second specific defense mechanism used by phobics to get the source outside of themselves and into the external world.

The neutral object chosen unconsciously is the one which can be easily avoided (the third defense mechanism) in day-to-day life, incontrast to the frightening object.

If the item is dogs, the individual avoids dogs. The end result is that the three combined defenses may eliminate the anxiety because the unacceptable or forbidden thought is re-repressed.

Freud's case of Little Hans is the model for the psychoanalytical understanding of phobias. Freud conceptualized Little Hans's fear of horses as resulting from unconscious oedipal fears. Little Hans denied these fears and projected them onto horses. Accordingly, symptoms of phobia are thought to be related to unresolved unconscious conflicts. The anxiety of the conflict is experienced, but the source of the anxiety is shifted onto an unrelated and harmless object, and the real source of anxiety is kept from consciousness.

Biologic Theories

Evidence suggests amygdala as the major mediator of the stress response, fear, and possibly also anxiety. Some evidence suggests dopaminergic, GABA and serotonrgic dysfunction in these areas may cause phobia (Kaplan and Saddock, 1999).

Twin studies suggest that specific phobia has the lowest genetic contribution of any of the anxiety disorders.

Phobias may have a genetic back up. For example, some individuals with blood-injection-injury phobias, which strongly clusters among biological relatives, may be genetically predisposed by vagal responses to certain stimuli.

Management

Pharmacotherapy

- SSRIs are the drug of choice—paroxetine is the most widely used. Fluoxetine and sertraline are also effective.
- Benzodiazepines—alprazolam (anti-phobic, anti-panic, and anti-anxiety) to reduce anticipatory anxiety.
- Drug treatments for specific phobia have consistently been shown to be less effective than behavioral treatments.
- β-blockers reduce some symptoms of sympathetic arousal during exposure to feared stimuli. However, they fail to decrease subjective fear.
- While benzodiazepines may facilitate approach to the feared stimuli, they may also reduce the efficacy of behavior therapies by inhibiting the experience of anxiety during exposure.
- β-blockers-propranolol has been found to effective in reducing autonomic symptoms.

Cognitive-behavioral Interventions

- Combining progressive relaxation and graduated imaginal exposure to the feared stimulus, systematic desensitization has been used.
- Systematic desensitization works by the principle of reciprocal inhibition, which asserts that the sympathetic response associated with anxiety is incompatible with, and thus inhibited by, the parasympathetic response that occurs during deep muscle relaxation.

Exposure

Prolonged and repeated *in vivo* exposure to feared stimuli is by far the most studied and effective form of treatment for specific phobia.

Cognitive restructuring—phobia-specific irrational thoughts may contribute to the development of the phobia, maintain avoidance behavior, and contribute to physiological symptoms. Cognitive restructuring treatments help patients to monitor irrational thoughts and change underlying beliefs, so that they are better able to enter feared situations.

OBSESSIVE COMPULSIVE DISORDER

An obsession is defined as

1. An idea, impulse or image which intrudes into conscious awareness repeatedly
2. It is recognized as an irrational (insight is present)

3. Patient tries to resist against it but is unable to
4. Failure to resist leads to marked distress.
   The important categories of obsessions are:
   - Fear of contamination (impurity, pollution, badness)
   - Orderliness of inanimate object
   - Doubts (worrying about whether one has omitted to do something)
   - Aggressive or fightening impulses
   - Recurrent sexual thoughts or images
   - An obsession is usually associated with a compulsion
     A compulsion is defines as:
     - A form of behavior which usually follows obsessions.
     - It is aimed at either preventing or neutralizing the distress or fear arising out of obsession.
     - Insight is present, so the patient realizes the irrationality of compulsion.
     - The behavior is performed with a sense of subjective compulsion (urge or impulse to act.)

Common compulsions are:
1. Washing/cleaning
2. Counting
3. Checking
4. Repeated actions
5. Making lists.

Compulsion may diminish the anxiety associated with obsessions.

Etiology

Behavioral Theory

Obsession: Conditioned stimuli to anxiety
Compulsion: Learned behavior which decrease the anxiety associated with obsession.
This decrease in anxiety positively reinforces the compulsive act and they become stable learned behaviors.

Biological Theory

- Secondary to basal ganglia lesion.
- Altered serotonin level, noradrenaline.
- Genetic: It can be transmitted genetically.
- EEG: Temporal lobe spikes and increased theta waves have been reported in sleep EEG of OCD subjects.

Clinical Syndroms

Washers

This is the commonest type. Here the obsession is of contamination with dirt, germs, body excretions. The compulsion is washing of hands or whole body repeatedly many times a day.

It usually spreads on to washing of cloths, washing of bathroom, bedroom, door knobs and personal articles gradually.

The person tries to avoid contamination but is unable to. So washing becomes a ritual.

Checkers

In this type, the person has multiple doubts. For example, the door has not been locked, kitchen gas has been left open, counting of money was not exact.

The compulsion of course is checking repeatedly to remove the doubt. Any attempt to stop the checking leads to mounting anxiety. Before one doubt has been cleared, other doubts may creep in.

Pure Obsessions

This syndrome is characterized by repetitive intrusive thoughts, impulses or images which are not associated with compulsive acts.
The content is usually sexual or aggressive in native.

Primary Obsessive Slowness

A relatively rare syndrome, it is characterized by severe obsessive ideas and/or extensive compulsive rituals, in the relative absence of manifested anxiety. This leads to marked slowness in daily activities.

Need for symmetry
- Persons suffering from an obsession about symmetry often report feeling acutely uncomfortable unless they perform certain tasks in a symmetrical or balanced manner, e.g. crossing one's legs to the right must be followed by crossing legs to the left.
- Scratching one side of the head must be followed by scratching the other.

Symptoms in Children
- Unusual behaviors in children that may be signs of OCD include.
- Avoidance of scissors or other sharp object. A child may be obsessed with fears of hurting herself or others.
- Chronic lateness. The child may be performing checking rituals. (repeatedly making sure all her school supplier are in her book bag).
- Daydreaming or preoccupation. The child may be counting or performing balancing rituals mentally.
- Spending long periods of time in the bathroom.

Treatment

1. Psychotherapy
   Supportive psychotherapy.

2. Behavior therapy
   Techniques used are thought stopping, response prevention, systematic desensitization, modeling, time out
3. Drugs:
   - Benzodiazepines (to control anxiety)
   - Anti-depressant—SSRI-flutetine.
   - TCA—clomipramine 75–300 mg/day
   - Anti-psychotic—haloperidol.
4. ECT
   In the presence of severe depression with OCD, ECT may be needed. ECT is particularly indicated when there is a risk of suicide and/or when there is a poor response to other modes of treatment. However, ECT is not the treatment of first choice is OCD.
5. Psychosurgery:
   - Stereotactic limbic leucotomy
   - Stereotactic sub-caudate leucotomy.

HYSTERICAL NEUROSIS (DISSOCIATIVE AND CONVERSION DISORDER)

This is derived from Greek word 'Hysteria' meaning womb or 'uterus'. Historically, it considered a female disorder. Freud used the word "conversion". Janet coined the term 'dissociation'.

Conversion Disorder

Unconscious process through which anxiety is converted into physical symptoms.

Feature

- Change physical functions
- Sudden onset
- Clear temporal relationship between stressor and development symptoms.
- Patient does not consciously produce symptoms.
- There is usually a secondary gain.
- Physical examination and investigation does not reveal any abnormality.

Symptoms

Physical (conversion) symptoms
The symptoms distribution is according to the patient's knowledge of nervous system.
Motor—paralysis, tremor, rigidity, abnormal gait, hysterial fits.
Sensory general—anesthesia, paresthesia, hyperalgesia pain.
Sensors special—visual difficulties, blindness, deafness, loss of taste, loss of smell.

Visceral—hiccough, vomiting, retention of urine, Constipation.
Others—respiratory problem, rapid heart rate, spasms in the body, redness of the eye, extreme salivation, clenching of the teeth.

Dissociative Disorder

This is an anxiety relieving hysterical problem. Here, the person dissociates or separates himself from the original self and acts in a new manner.

Mental (Dissociates) Symptoms

- Dissociative (hysterical) amnesia: Sudden inability to recall important personal information
  Types:
  - Circumscribed amnesia: Inability to recall all the personal events during a circumscribed period of time.
  - Selective amnesia: Inability to recall only some selective personal events.
  - Continuous amnesia: Inability to recall all personal events following the stressful events till the present time.
  - Generalized amnesia: Inability to recalls the personal events of the whole life.

  During the amnesia period, there may be slight clouding of consciousness.
- Dissociative fugue: It is wandering state. Patient assume new identity and inability to recall the past.
- Hysterical trance: It is ritualistic dance like behavior during the religious ceremonies. People feel that a spirit has entered her body and believe that she has the power to heal the sick and communicate with the dead or to predict the future.
- Hysterical possession state: It is culture-bound syndrome. The patient behave as if she is possessed by a God.
- Multiple personality: Transition from one personality to another is sudden and often associated with psychological stress.
- Hysterical pseudo dementia (Ganser's syndrome): The answers are wrong but show that the person understands the nature of question asked. Commonly found in prisons in mates.

Treatment

- Behavior therapy: Aversion therapy.
- Psychotherapy with abreaction: Abreaction is bringing to conscious awareness, thoughts, affects and memories for the first time. This may be achieved by: Hypnosis, Free association, Nalco analysis.
- Support psychotherapy
- Drug therapy
- Short-term benzodiazepines.

POST-TRAUMATIC STRESS DISORDER

Actually, the disorder arises when people are exposed to severe stressful, life-threatening situations in which they perceive that they have no control over the outcome. Those affected have flashbacks about the situation in which they were helpless, nightmares, difficulty sleeping, and find it impossible to put the situation behind them and get on with their lives. Situations inducing the disorder include military combat, natural disasters (e.g. being caught in an earthquake), accidents (e.g. a plane crash or train wreck) and being taken hostage, among others.

THE SOMATOFORM DISORDERS

"Soma" means "body," so these are disorders with some obvious connection to the state of the body.
- Hypochondriasis—You are probably more familiar with the label for the person: "hypochondriac". This is someone who is perpetually convinced that he or she has some dread disease which, if not treated promptly, is going to lead to their demise. If their own diagnosis is not confirmed by the doctor, hypochontriacs are likely to ask for a second opinion or to decide that, well, if it is not THIS, then surely it must be THAT. The disorder may be maintained by a strong fear of death, although being the center of attention and concern of physicians, friends, and others can provide its own source of motivation.

Management in Neurotic Patient

- Maintain a calm, non-threatening manner
- Reassure the patient by physical presence of nurse
- Use simple words, spoke calmly and clearly
- keep immediate surroundings low in stimuli
- Teach the signs and symptoms of anxiety provoking situation
- Explore the cause of threat
- Discuss reality of situation
- Selection of alternative coping strategies
- Provide relaxation techniques
- Assess patient's mood
- Encourage the independency by positive reinforcement
- Do not abruptly stop the behavior
- Provide structured schedule of activities
- Set up limit for the behavior
- Reassure the relatives (There is no organic base for the symptoms. It is not advisable to tell the relatives that she is in acting or malingering).
- The nurse should give an impression to the patient that she has no problem
- The nurse should give an impression to the patient that she is very concerned, thereby establishing rapport and gaining the patients confidence
- Ventilate patient feeling
- Administer medication as tranquilizers.

PREMENSTRUAL SYNDROME (PMS)

Premenstrual syndrome (PMS) is a group of symptoms linked to the menstrual cycle. PMS symptoms occur 1 to 2 weeks before your period (menstruation or monthly bleeding) starts. The symptoms usually go away after you start bleeding. PMS can affect menstruating women of any age and the effect is different for each woman. For some people, PMS is just a monthly bother. For others, it may be so severe that it makes it hard to even get through the day. PMS goes away when your monthly periods stop, such as when you get pregnant or go through menopause.

Causes

The causes of PMS are not clear, but several factors may be involved. Changes in hormones during the menstrual cycle seem to be an important cause. These changing hormone levels may affect some women more than others. Chemical changes in the brain may also be involved. Stress and emotional problems, such as depression, do not seem to cause PMS, but they may make it worse. Some other possible causes include:
- Low levels of vitamins and minerals
- Eating a lot of salty foods, which may cause you to retain (keep) fluid
- Drinking alcohol and caffeine, which may alter your mood and energy level.

Symptoms

PMS often includes both physical and emotional symptoms, such as: Acne, swollen or tender breasts, feeling tired, trouble sleeping, upset stomach, bloating, constipation or diarrhea, headache or backache, appetite changes or food cravings, joint or muscle pain, trouble with concentration or memory, tension, irritability, mood swings, or crying spells, anxiety or depression.

Symptoms vary from woman to woman.

PMS occurs more often in women who:
- Are between their late 20s and early 40s
- Have at least 1 child
- Have a family history of depression
- Have a past medical history of either postpartum depression or a mood disorder.

Treatment

Many things have been tried to ease the symptoms of PMS. No treatment works for every woman. You may need to try different ones to see what works for you. Some treatment options include:
- Lifestyle changes
- Medications
- Alternative therapies.

Lifestyle Changes

If your PMS is not so bad that you need to see a doctor, some lifestyle changes may help you feel better. Below are some steps you can take that may help ease your symptoms.
- Exercise regularly. Each week, you should get:
Two hours and 30 minutes of moderate-intensity physical activity;
One hour and 15 minutes of vigorous-intensity aerobic physical activity; or
a combination of moderate and vigorous-intensity activity; and
muscle-strengthening activities on 2 or more days.
- Eat healthy foods, such as fruits, vegetables, and whole grains.
- Avoid salt, sugary foods, caffeine, and alcohol, especially when you are having PMS symptoms.
- Get enough sleep. Try to get about 8 hours of sleep each night.
- Find healthy ways to cope with stress. Talk to your friends, exercise, or write in a journal. Some women also find yoga, massage, or relaxation therapy helpful.
- Do not smoke.

Medications

Over-the-counter pain relievers may help ease physical symptoms, such as cramps, headaches, backaches, and breast tenderness. These include:
- Ibuprofen (for instance, Advil, Motrin, Midol Cramp)
- Ketoprofen (for instance, Orudis KT)
- Naproxen (for instance, Aleve)
- Aspirin.

In more severe cases of PMS, prescription medicines may be used to ease symptoms. One approach has been to use drugs that stop ovulation, such as birth control pills. Women on the pill report fewer PMS symptoms, such as cramps and headaches, as well as lighter periods.

Alternative Therapies

Certain vitamins and minerals have been found to help relieve some PMS symptoms. These include: Folic acid (400 micrograms)
- Calcium with vitamin D (see chart below for amounts)
- Magnesium (400 milligrams)
- Vitamin B-6 (50 to 100 mg)
- Vitamin E (400 international units).

Some women find their PMS symptoms relieved by taking supplements such as:
- Black cohosh
- Chasteberry
- Evening primrose oil.

Talk with your doctor before taking any of these products. Many have not been proven to work and they may interact with other medicines you are taking.

HYPERVENTILATION SYNDROME

Hyperventilation syndrome is a nonmedical cause of shortness of breath. Hyperventilation syndrome is very scary, but not life-threatening.

Causes of Hyperventilation Syndrome

The term hyperventilation syndrome evolved from the more descriptive *psychogenic hyperventilation syndrome*, which indicates a psychosomatic cause for the hyperventilation. Basically, that means there is usually some sort of behavioral or emotional reason for the hyperventilation. In most cases, hyperventilation goes hand-in-hand with anxiety or panic disorders. Many of the symptoms of hyperventilation syndrome appear during what are commonly called panic attacks.

There are other, more serious, medical conditions that may lead to hyperventilation. The most serious is related to an increase of pressure inside the skull (intracranial pressure). The increased pressure pushes the brain through the foramen magnum, the opening in the base of the skull where the spinal cord exits. This is called herniation of the brain and leads to neurogenic hyperventilation syndrome, an involuntary reaction of the respiratory centers in the brain to increases in pressure.

Recognizing Hyperventilation Syndrome

If a victim with rapid, shallow breathing has the ability to become more calm and slow his or her breathing, it may be hyperventilation syndrome. A behavioral cause of hyperventilation can be overcome, a medical cause of rapid breathing probably cannot. Treating hyperventilation syndrome often distinguishes the condition from other causes of shortness of breath as well as treats it.

Never assume a victim is suffering from hyperventilation syndrome. Always assess victims for other causes of shortness of breath first. It is important to note that hyperventilation syndrome patients must be conscious and able to communicate. Unconscious or unresponsive victims are likely not suffering from hyperventilation syndrome.

Hyperventilation Symptoms: The Nijmegen Questionnaire

Developed to screen patients complaining of shortness of breath for possible hyperventilation syndrome, the Nijmegen questionnaire identifies several signs and symptoms of hyperventilation syndrome. Correctly using this screening tool requires a clinical background, especially since many of the screening questions could be symptoms of much more serious medical conditions.

Of the hyperventilation syndrome symptoms and signs listed in the Nijmegen questionnaire, there are several that are distinctly related to hyperventilation syndrome. These signs and symptoms are strong indicators of hyperventilation syndrome, especially if the victim has several of them:
- Tense feeling
- Dizziness

- Fast or deep breathing
- Tingling in fingers and hands
- Stiffness or cramps in fingers and hands
- Tightness around the mouth
- Cold hands or feet
- Palpitations in the chest
- Anxiety.

Despite their relationship to hyperventilation syndrome, each of these signs and symptoms could also be related to other medical conditions. Always assume the worst possible scenario first, then proceed to less serious conditions, in order to identify the cause of shortness of breath.

IRRITABLE BOWEL SYNDROME (IBS)

Irritable bowel syndrome (IBS) is a "syndrome," meaning a group of symptoms. The most common symptoms of IBS are abdomenal pain or discomfort often reported as cramping, bloating, gas, diarrhea, and/or constipation. IBS affects the colon or large bowel, which is the part of the digestive tract that stores stool.

IBS is not a disease. It is a functional disorder, meaning that the bowel does not work, or function, correctly.

Causes

The nerves and muscles in the bowel appear to be extrasensitive in people with IBS. Muscles may contract too much when you eat. These contractions can cause cramping and diarrhea during or shortly after a meal. Or the nerves may react when the bowel stretches, causing cramping or pain.

IBS can be painful. But it does not damage the colon or other parts of the digestive system. IBS does not lead to other health problems.

Symptoms of IBS

The main symptoms of IBS are:
- Abdominal pain or discomfort in the abdomen, often relieved by or associated with a bowel movement
- Chronic diarrhea, constipation, or a combination of both.

Other symptoms are:
- Whitish mucus in the stool
- A swollen or bloated abdomen
- The feeling that you have not finished a bowel movement.

Women with IBS often have more symptoms during their menstrual periods.

Medical Tests for IBS

In addition to a physical exam and blood tests, the following tests might be done to diagnose IBS:

- **Lower gastrointestinal (GI) series.** This test uses X-rays to diagnose problems in the large intestine. It is also called a barium enema X-ray. Before you have the X-ray, the doctor will put barium into your large intestine through the anus—the opening where stool leaves the body. Barium is a thick liquid that makes your intestines show up better on the X-ray.
- **Colonoscopy.** For this test the doctor inserts a long, thin tube, called a colonoscope, into your anus and up into your colon. The tube has a light and tiny lens on the end. The doctor can view the inside of your colon on a big television screen. In some cases, a shorter tube, called a flexible sigmoidoscope, is used to look at just the lower portion of the colon.

Treatment

IBS has no cure, but you can do things to relieve symptoms. Treatment may involve:
- Diet changes
- Medicine
- Stress relief.

Diet Changes

Some foods and drinks make IBS worse.
Foods and drinks that may cause or worsen symptoms include:
- Fatty foods, like french fries
- Milk products, like cheese or ice cream
- Chocolate
- Alcohol
- Caffeinated drinks, like coffee and some sodas
- Carbonated drinks, like soda.

These foods may make IBS worse.
To find out which foods are a problem, keep a diary that tracks
- What you eat during the day
- What symptoms you have
- When symptoms occur
- What foods always make you feel sick.

Some Foods make IBS Better

Fiber may reduce the constipation associated with IBS because it makes stool soft and easier to pass. However, some people with IBS who have more sensitive nerves may feel a bit more abdominal discomfort after adding more fiber to their diet. Fiber is found in foods such as breads, cereals, beans, fruits, and vegetables.

Add foods with fiber to your diet a little at a time to let your body get used to them. Too much fiber at once can cause gas, which can trigger symptoms in a person with IBS.

Eat Small Meals

Large meals can cause cramping and diarrhea in people with IBS. If this happens to you, try eating four or five small meals a day instead of less-frequent big meals.

Medicine

Laxatives treat constipation. Many kinds of laxatives are available. Your doctor can help you find the laxative that is right for you.
- Antispasmodics control spasms in the colon and help ease abdominal pain.
- Antidepressants, even in lower doses than are used for treating depression, can help people with IBS. They can help reduce the abdominal discomfort or pain associated with IBS and, depending on the type chosen, may help the diarrhea or constipation.

Another drug is sometimes prescribed for the treatment of IBS. Alosetron hydrochloride (Lotronex) is for women with severe IBS whose main symptom is diarrhea. Because it can cause serious side effects, Lotronex is only used if other medicines do not work.

Chapter 7

Psychoactive Substance Use Disorder

PSYCHOACTIVE DRUGS

The term 'psychoactive drug' is used to describe any chemical substance that affects mood, perception or consciousness as a result of changes in the functioning of the nervous system (brain and spinal cord).

Psychoactive drugs are divided into 3 groups:
- Depressants: They slow down the central nervous system; for example: tranquillisers, alcohol, petrol, heroin and other opiates, cannabis (in low doses).
- Stimulants: They excite the nervous system; for example: Nicotine, amphetamines, cocaine, caffeine.
- Hallucinogens: They distort how things are perceived; for example: LSD, mescaline, 'magic mushrooms', cannabis (in high doses).

Effects of Using Drugs

A drug can have psychological, emotional and physical effects and can change the behavior of the person taking the drug. These behavioral changes are not the same for everyone. The effect of any drug will depend on:

The drug: What effect it has on the central nervous system; the amount taken; how it is taken; how often; for how long; if it is taken with other drugs.

The person: Age, weight, sex, tolerance, past experiences, mood, personality, the expectations and what the person wants to happen from using the drug.

The environment: What the community or society expects, allows and excuses as a result of using the drug; the place; the presence of other people; noise levels, and so forth (adapted from Saunders and O'Connor, 1994; Matthews 1997:24; Keenan in Hamilton et al 1998:64).

Reason for People Use Drugs

There are many reasons why people use drugs. Can you think of some reasons and list them? Compare them with the following most common reasons people give for using drugs:
- For pleasure—they like the feeling the drug gives
- Because friends and family use them
- Because they like the 'taste'
- To relieve tension and relax

- To be part of a religious ceremony
- Because they are lonely
- To relieve boredom
- For pain relief
- To help cope with problems and forget worries
- Because they have grown dependent on the drug
- Because they feel ill if they stop
- To do things that they usually could not or would not do—it gives them courage.

In remote Aboriginal communities and in town camps, life can be really tough, especially for young people. There is often little to do. People can feel caught between what their parents and elders say is important and the pressures and promises that western culture seems to offer. Community stress, boredom, frustration and peer pressure can draw people into drug using lifestyles.

The following diagram shows the three major influences on an individual's decisions about drug use. Addressing drug-related harm needs to consider the links between these different factors.

Some Useful Terms and Concepts

Abstinence

The word 'abstinence' is used when people decide not to use a drug or to stop taking a drug or substance at all times and under all circumstances. People who abstain usually do not intend to use the drug again.

Addiction, Addictive Behavior

Addiction to a drug means that the person:
- Has a strong desire or compulsion to use the drug (cannot think about anything else)
- Finds it difficult to control the drug using behavior
- Is uncomfortable or distressed if the drug taking is prevented or stops (withdrawal symptoms)
- Keeps using the drug, even when it is causing problems.

Sometimes this word is used in the same way as drug dependence. The problem with using the word 'addiction' is that people are often labelled as 'junkies' or 'drug addicts'. This term can make us think of them as criminals, dangerous and generally unpleasant people. It also suggests that they are unable to control their lives or change drug taking patterns.

Binge Drinking

- Binge drinking refers to the rapid consumption of alcohol over a short period of time to the point of intoxication. There are two forms of binge drinking:
    - The consumption of five or more drinks in one drinking session
    - Heavy and continuous drinking over a number of days or weeks.

Detoxification

The process by which an individual is withdrawn from the effects of a pychoactive substance. Typically, the individual is clinically intoxicated or already in withdrawal at the outset of detoxification. Detoxification may or may not involve the administration of medication.

Drug Abuse

This term is often used to describe drug use that causes harm. The problem with using this term is that it can create negative feelings or attitudes toward the user and is not a recommended term to use.

Drug Misuse

This term is also used to describe harmful or inappropriate use of drugs. It is the preferred term because it does not have the same negative meanings about the user.

Drug Dependence

Drug dependence occurs when a drug becomes central to a person's thoughts, emotions and activities. Using the drug takes on a higher priority than many other things in life and the person may neglect other responsibilities.

Being dependent makes it hard for people to stop or even cut down on the drug. They may want to take the drug continually for its effects or to avoid the discomfort and distress of not having it (withdrawal).

Harmful Use

This term describes drug use that causes damage to either mental or physical health. It can also refer to the harm caused to the drug user's family or community in general.

Intoxication

People are said to be intoxicated when they use an amount of a substance that produces noticeable changes in their behavior.

Recreational or Social Use

Sometimes people use a drug or drugs on a casual basis to enhance socializing or to increase their enjoyment of leisure and recreational activities.

Tolerance

If a person repeatedly takes a drug, the person's body becomes used to working with a certain level of the drug in the bloodstream. The person's body adapts to the presence of the drug; that is, the person develops a tolerance to the drug. The person then has to increase his or her intake of the drug to get the desired effect, for example, to feel 'high'.

Tolerance can develop to most drugs if they are used on a regular basis. People who regularly use alcohol, tobacco, coffee and tea will have developed a tolerance to them. They may feel unwell when they stop taking the drug.

Withdrawal

Dependence, both physical and psychological, results from regular use of some drugs. When a person stops taking the drug, he or she may experience certain unpleasant physical and mental effects. This group of effects is referred to as 'withdrawal symptoms'. They are different for each drug. When a person is experiencing these symptoms, the person is said to be 'in withdrawal'.

ALCOHOL USE DISORDER

Alcohol is produced by fermenting the starch or sugar in fruits and grains. Alcoholic drinks have different amounts of alcohol in them—beer is about 5% alcohol, wine is usually 12–15% alcohol, and hard liquor is about 45% alcohol. Common facts about alcohol are given in Table 7.1.

Table 7.1: Facts about alcohol

Three important facts about alcohol
1. Alcohol contains a lot of empty calories without any vitamins and minerals.
2. Many people think that alcohol is a stimulant. This is not true. Alcohol is a depressant.
3. Some users become dependent on alcohol such dependence causes serious problems related to occupation, family, finance, society.

Alternative Names

Beer consumption; wine consumption; hard liquor consumption.

The Immediate Effect of Alcohol

Alcohol is absorbed into your bloodstream quickly. The absorption rate depends on the amount and type of food in your stomach. For example, high carbohydrate and high fat foods lessen the absorption rates. A carbonated alcoholic drink, like champagne, will be absorbed faster.

The effects of alcohol may appear within 10 minutes and peak at approximately 40 to 60 minutes. Alcohol remains in the bloodstream until it is broken down by the liver. If a person consumes alcohol at a faster rate than it can be broken down by the liver, the blood alcohol concentration level rises.

Each state has its own legal definition for alcohol intoxication, which is defined by blood alcohol concentration. The legal limit usually falls between 0.08 and 0.10 in most states. Different levels lead to different effects:
- 0.05 reduced inhibitions
- 0.10 slurred speech
- 0.20 euphoria and motor impairment
- 0.30 confusion
- 0.40 stupor
- 0.50 coma
- 0.60 respiratory paralysis and death.

Alcohol depresses your breathing rate, heart rate, and the control mechanisms in your brain. The effects include:

- Less ability to drive and perform complex tasks
- Reduced inhibitions, which may lead to embarrassing behavior
- Reduced attention span
- Impaired short-term memory
- Impaired motor coordination
- Prolonged reaction time
- Less rapid thought processes.
- If a pregnant woman drinks, alcohol can adversely affect the developing fetus causing birth defects or fetal alcohol syndrome (a devastating disorder marked by mental retardation and behavioral problems). Table 7.2 explain myths about alcoholism and alcohol abuse.

Table 7.2: Myths about alcoholism and alcohol abuse
Five myths about alcoholism and alcohol abuse
Myth #1: I can stop drinking anytime I want to.
Maybe you can; more likely, you can not. Either way, it is just an excuse to keep drinking. The truth is, you do not want to stop. Telling yourself you can quit makes you feel in control, despite all evidence to the contrary and no matter the damage it is doing.
Myth #2: My drinking is my problem. I am the one it hurts, so no one has the right to tell me to stop.
It is true that the decision to quit drinking is up to you. But you are deceiving yourself if you think that your drinking hurts no one else but you. Alcoholism affects everyone around you—especially the people closest to you. Your problem is their problem.
Myth #3: I do not drink every day, so I can't be an alcoholic OR I only drink wine or beer, so I can not be an alcoholic.
Alcoholism is NOT defined by what you drink, when you drink it, or even how much you drink. It is the EFFECTS of your drinking that define a problem. If your drinking is causing problems in your home or work life, you have a drinking problem and may be an alcoholic—whether you drink daily or only on the weekends, down shots of tequila or stick to wine, drink three bottles of beers a day or three bottles of whiskey.
Myth #4: I am not an alcoholic because I have a job and I am doing okay.
You do not have to be homeless and drinking out of a brown paper bag to be an alcoholic. Many alcoholics are able to hold down jobs, get through school, and provide for their families. Some are even able to excel. But just because you are a high-functioning alcoholic does not mean you are not putting yourself or others in danger. Over time, the effects will catch up with you.
Myth #5: Drinking is not a "real" addiction like drug abuse.
Alcohol is a drug, and alcoholism is every bit as damaging as drug addiction. Alcohol addiction causes changes in the body and brain, and long-term alcohol abuse can have devastating effects on your health, your career, and your relationships. Alcoholics go through physical withdrawal when they stop drinking, just like drug users do when they quit.

Health Risks

Alcohol increases the risks of:
- Motor vehicle accidents
- Falls, drownings and other accidents
- Suicide and homicide

- Increased risk for homicide
- Risky sex behaviors, unplanned or unwanted pregnancy, and sexually transmitted diseases (STDs)
- Fetal alcohol syndrome if a pregnant woman drinks
- Alcoholism or alcohol dependence
- Chronic liver disease
- Head, neck, stomach, and breast cancers.

Dependence Syndrome

Individuals who consume alcohol (or live with individuals who consume alcohol) may want to seek help for themselves or loved ones if the following occur in association with drinking behavior:
- Driving citations or accidents (DUI)
- Decreased interest or performance levels at work, school
- Increased absenteeism from work, school
- Increased social isolation
- Increased tolerance to amount of alcohol consumed: More alcohol is needed to produce the same effect
- Inability to decrease or stop alcohol consumption
- Signs of withdrawal, such as tremors, appear when attempting to stop
- Defensive or hostile about personal alcohol use
- Lying or being secretive about alcohol use
- Neglecting appearance
- Neglecting proper nutrition
- Involved in violence, either as perpetrator or victim.

It is also important to remember that some individuals are at higher risk for alcoholism due to a family history of alcoholism, stressful lifestyles, peer or cultural influences, and psychological factors such as anxiety, depression, or even low self-esteem.

Complications of Alcohol Dependence

Medical Complications

- Gastrointestinal system
    - Fatly liver, cirrhosis of liver, hepatitis, liver cell carcinoma
    - Gastritis, peptic ulcer, carcinoma esophagus
    - Malabsorption syndrome
    - Pancreatitis: acute and chronic
- Central nervous system
    - Peripheral neuropathy
    - Alcoholic jealously
    - Suicide
    - Head injury and fractions

- Miscellaneous
  - Palmar erythema
  - Fetal alcohol syndrome (craniofacial anomalies, growth retardation, major organ system malformation)
  - Alcoholic hypoglycemia and ketoacidosis
  - Cardiomyopath
  - Anemia, thrombocytopenia, vitamin K factor deficiency hemolytic anemia
  - Accidental hypothermia
  - Pseudo-cushing's syndrome, infertility, amenorrhea decreased testosterone and increased LH levels.
  - Risk for coronary artery disease
  - Malnutrition.

Social Complication

- Accidents
- Criminality
- Marital disharmony
- Financial difficulties
- Divorce
- Occupational problem

Neuropsychiatic Complications of Chronic Alcohol Use

1. Wernicke's encephalopthy:
   This is an acute reaction to severe thiamin deficiency. The onset occurs after a period of persistent vomiting. The important clinical signs are:
   i. Ocular signs: Coarse nystagmus, ophthalmoplegia with bilateral external rectus paralysis occur early. Papillary irregularities, retinal hemorrhages and papilledema can occur, causing impairment of vision.
   ii. Higher mental function disturbance: Disorientation, recent memory disturbances, poor attention span and distractibility are common. Apathy is an early symptom.
2. Korsakoff's psychosis (severe thiamin deficiency):
   Korsakoff's psychosis presents as an amnestic syndrome, characterized by gross memory disturbances with confabulation. Insight is often impaired.
3. Marchiafava Bignami disease:
   This is a rare disorder characterized by disorientation, epilepsy, ataxia, dysarthria, hallucinations, and spastic limb paralysis and personality and intellectual deterioration.

Others:
Alcoholic dementia, cerebella degeneration, peripheral neuropathy, central pontine myelinosis.

For detection of problem drinkers in the community, several screening instruments are available. Michigan alcoholism screening test (MAST) is frequently used for this purpose. While CAGE questionnaire is the easiest to be administered (It takes only about 1–2 minutes).

The CAGE questionnaire consists of 4 questions:
1. Have you ever had to cut down on alcohol.
2. Have you ever been Annoyed by peoples criticism of alcoholism.
3. Have you ever felt guilty about drinking.
4. Have you ever needed eye opener drink (early morning drink).

A score of 2 or more identifies problem drinkers.

Medical Treatment

It consists of detoxification and treatment of alcohol dependence.

Detoxification

This is the treatment of alcohol withdrawal symptoms. The best way to stop alcohol is to stop it suddenly.

Aim: The aim of detoxification is the symptomatic management of the emergent withdrawal symptoms.

Drug of choice: Chlordiazepoxide 80–200 mg/day, diazepam 40–80 mg/day.
The dosage should be decreased everyday before being stopped, usually on the 10th day.
Vitamin B 100 mg IV BD for 5 days followed by oral vitamin B1 for atleast 6 months.
Antacids.

Treatment of Alcohol Dependence

Behavior therapy: The most commonly used behavior therapy are relaxation technique, self-assertive skill training, self-control, positive reinforcements.
    Films of their own drinking pattern is taken and are shown to them.
The therapy helps to modify the behavior pattern and increases the coping ability and assertiveness in life.

Psychotherapy: Supportive psychotherapy and individual psychotherapy have been used.

Deterrent agents: The deterrent agents are also called alcohol sensitizing drugs.
Drug: Disulfiram (tetraethyl thiuram disulfide):
    250–500 mg/day in the first weak
    250 mg/day maintenance dose.
Action
When alcohol is ingested by a person who is on disulfiram, alcohol-derived acetaldehyde cannot be oxidized to acetate and this leads to an accumulation of acetaldehyde in blood. This is called disulfiram ethanol reaction (DER).

The onset of the reaction occur within 30 minitus and subsides usually within 2 hours of ingestion of alcohol. DER is characterized by flushing, tachycardia, hypotension, tachypnea, palpation, headache, sweating, nausea, vomiting, giddiness and anxiety.

In severe DER patient may face shock, myocardial infarction, convulsion, confusion and coma.

Contraindications of disulfiram use : First trimester of pregnancy, coronary artery disease, liver failure, chronic renal failure, peripheral neuropathy, muscle disease, history of psychosis in past.

Other deterrent
- Citrated calcium carbimide (CCC)
- Antipsychotics, antidepressants
- Lithium, carbamazepine
- Narcotics.

OPIOIDS AND RELATED DISORDER

Definition

Opioids are a class of drugs that include both natural and synthetic substances. The natural opioids (referred to as opiates) include opium and morphine. Heroin, the most abused opioid, is synthesized from opium. Other synthetics (only made in laboratories) and commonly prescribed for pain, such as cough suppressants, or as anti-diarrhea agents, include codeine, oxycodone (Oxycontin), meperidine (Demerol), fentanyl (Sublimaze), hydromorphone (Dilaudid), methadone and propoxyphene (Darvon). Heroin is usually injected, either intravenously (into a vein) or subcutaneously (under the skin), but can be smoked or used intranasally (i.e. snorted). Other opioids are either injected or taken orally.

Opioid Dependence

Dependence on opioids involves significant physiological and psychological changes, which make it extremely difficult for an individual to stop using the opioids. Recurrent use of opioids causes actual changes in how the brain functions. An individual who is addicted to opioids cannot simply just stop using, despite significant negative consequences related to their use. Marital difficulties, including divorce, unemployment, and drug-related legal problems are often associated with opioid dependence. People dependent on opioids often plan their day around obtaining and using opioids.

Opioid Abuse

People who abuse opioids typically use them less frequently than those who are dependent on opioids. However, despite less frequent use, an individual with opioid abuse suffers negative consequences. For example, while intoxicated on opioids, an individual may get arrested for their behavior.

Opioid intoxication

An individual who uses opioids typically experiences drowsiness (nodding off), mood changes, a feeling of heaviness, dry mouth, itching, and slurred speech. Individuals who use heroin intravenously describe an intense euphoria (or rush), a floating feeling, and total indifference to pain. Symptoms of intoxication usually last several hours. Severe intoxication from an overdose of opioids is life-threatening because breathing may stop.

Opioid Withdrawal

Tolerance to opioids occurs quickly. Regular users of opioids take doses that would kill someone who has never used before. After regular use, the human body adapts to the regular presence of the drug and the person only feels "normal" when they have opioids in their system. Therefore, when an opioid-dependent individual stops using opioids abruptly, he or she will experience withdrawal symptoms. Withdrawal symptoms from heroin usually begin six to eight hours after last use and peak after two days. Acute withdrawal typically lasts no more than seven to ten days, but some symptoms of withdrawal (such as craving, insomnia, anxiety, lack of interest) can last six months or longer. Although withdrawal is very uncomfortable, it is not life-threatening unless there is an underlying medical condition, such as heart disease. In addition to physical withdrawal, "psychological withdrawal" often occurs. The individual who is dependent on opioids has difficulty imagining living without the drug, since they were dependent on it to function. This is similar to how someone addicted to nicotine may feel after giving up cigarettes.

Treatments

Opioid Dependence

Because opioid-related disorders are complex, multiple treatment approaches are often necessary. Generally, the more treatment (a combination of medication, individual therapy, and so, for example) if help group and longer the treatment (i.e. at least three months), the better the outcomes. There are a wide variety of treatment options, both inpatient or residential and outpatient:
- Methadone maintenance treatment: Methadone is a long-acting opioid that is generally administered in an outpatient setting (a methadone maintenance clinic). The methadone prevents the individual from experiencing opioid withdrawal, reduces opioid craving, and enables the individual to have access to other services (such as individual counseling, medical services, and HIV-prevention education). A proper dose of methadone also prevents the individual from getting "high" from heroin. Methadone maintenance therapy can decrease criminal activity, decrease HIV-risk behaviors, and increase stability of employment. Low-dose methadone maintenance treatment is preferable for pregnant individuals who would otherwise use illicit opioids. A

longer-acting alternative to methadone is levo-alphacetylmethadol (LAAM). Individuals receiving the proper doses of LAAM only need to take it three times per week, instead of every day as with methadone.

- Opioid antagonist treatment: An opioid antagonist is a medication that blocks the effects of opioids. Treatment with an antagonist, usually naltrexone (Trexan), typically takes place on an outpatient basis following an inpatient medical detoxification from opioids. The effects of taking any opioids are blocked by the naltrexone and prevent the individual from getting "high," thereby discouraging individuals from seeking opioids. By itself, this treatment is suitable for individuals highly motivated to discontinue opioid use. However, antagonists can be used in addition to other treatment modalities or with individuals who have been abstinent for some time but fear a relapse.
- Opioid agonist-antagonist treatment: An opioid agonist is a drug that has a similar action to morphine. Buprenorphine (Buprenex) is an example of an opioid agonist-antagonist, which means it acts as both an agonist (having some morphine-like action) and antagonist (it blocks the effects of additional opioids). Buprenorphine has been shown to effectively reduce opioid use. It is also being studied for opioid detoxification.
- Outpatient drug-free treatment: These are outpatient treatment approaches that do not include medications. There are a number of different types of programs ranging from simple drug education to intensive outpatient programs that offer most of the services of an inpatient setting. Some programs may specialize in treating specific groups of people who are opioid-dependent (those with co-occurring mental disorders, for example).
- Residential or inpatient treatment: These include inpatient rehabilitation programs (usually 7 to 30 days in length) and long-term residential programs (such as therapeutic communities). Rehabilitation programs provide an inpatient atmosphere following detoxification and usually offer individual and group counseling as well as medical services. Therapeutic communities are designed to be more than six months long and are highly structured. The primary focus is on resocializing the individual to a drug-free and crime-free lifestyle.
- Individualized drug counseling: Individual counseling is often a part of a methadone maintenance program or inpatient rehabilitation program. The primary focus is on helping the individual learn strategies to reduce or stop their opioid use and learn coping mechanisms to maintain abstinence. Twelve-step participation is encouraged and referrals for medical, psychiatric, employment, or other services are made as necessary.
- Supportive-expressive psychotherapy: This type of individual psychotherapy may be a part of a methadone maintenance program or offered alone. The focus of this type of therapy is to help individuals feel comfortable talking about themselves, work on relationship issues, and solve problems without resorting to opioids or other drugs.

- Self-help groups: Narcotics Anonymous (NA) is a twelve-step group based on the same model as Alcoholics Anonymous. This self-help group can provide social support to an individual in the process of reducing or stopping opioid use. Participation in NA is often encouraged or is a required component of other types of treatment for opioid dependence. Nar-Anon is a group for family members and friends of opioid-dependent individuals.

COCAINE AND RELATED DISORDER

Definition

Cocaine is extracted from the coca plant, which grows in Central and South America. The substance is processed into many forms for use as an illegal drug of abuse. Cocaine is dangerously addictive, and users of the drug experience a "high"—a feeling of euphoria or intense happiness, along with hypervigilance, increased sensitivity, irritablity or anger, impaired judgment, and anxiety.

Forms of the Drug

In its most common form, cocaine is a whitish crystalline powder that produces feelings of euphoria when ingested. In powder form, cocaine is known by such street names as "coke," "blow," "C," "flake," "snow" and "toot." It is most commonly inhaled or "snorted." It may also be dissolved in water and injected.

Crack is a form of cocaine that can be smoked and that produces an immediate, more intense, and more short-lived high. It comes in off-white chunks or chips called "rocks".

In addition to their stand-alone use, both cocaine and crack are often mixed with other substances. Cocaine may be mixed with methcathinone to create a "wildcat." Cigars may be hollowed out and filled with a mixture of crack and marijuana. Either cocaine or crack used in conjunction with heroin is called a "speedball." Cocaine used together with alcohol represents the most common fatal two-drug combination.

Cocaine-induced Disorders

Cocaine intoxication: Cocaine intoxication occurs after recent cocaine use. The person experiences a feeling of intense happiness, hypervigilance, increased sensitivity, irritability or anger, with impaired judgment, and anxiety. The intoxication impairs the person's ability to function at work, school, or in social situations. Two or more of the following symptoms are present immediately after the use of the cocaine—enlarged pupils, elevated heart rate, elevated or lowered blood pressure, chills and increased sweating, nausea or vomiting, weight loss, agitation or slowed movements, weak muscles, chest pain, coma, confusion, irregular heartbeat, depressed respiration, seizures, odd postures and odd movements.

Cocaine withdrawal: As mentioned, withdrawal symptoms develop within hours or days after cocaine use that has been heavy and prolonged and then abruptly stopped. The symptoms include irritable mood and two or more of the following symptoms—fatigue, nightmares, difficulty sleeping or too much sleep, elevated appetite, agitation (restlessness), or slowed physical movements.

Symptoms

The following list is a summary of the acute (short-term) physical and psychological effects of cocaine on the body: blood vessels constrict, elevated heart rate, elevated blood pressure, a feeling of intense happiness, elevated energy level, a state of increased alertness and sensory sensitivity, elevated anxiety, panic attacks, elevated self-esteem, diminished appetite, spontaneous ejaculation and heightened sexual arousal and psychosis (loss of contact with reality).

Treatments

Psychotherapy: A wide range of behavioral interventions have been successfully used to treat cocaine addiction. However, the approach used must be tailored to the specific needs of each individual patient.

Contingency management rewards drug abstinence (confirmed by urine testing) with points or vouchers which patients can exchange for such things as an evening out or membership in a gym. Cognitive-behavioral therapy helps users learn to recognize and avoid situations most likely to lead to cocaine use and to develop healthier ways to cope with stressful situations.

Supportive therapy helps patients to modify their behavior by preventing relapse by taking actions such as staying away from drug-using friends and from neighborhoods or situations where cocaine is abundant.

Self-help groups like Narcotics Anonymous (NA) or Cocaine Anonymous (CA) are helpful for many recovering substance abusers. CA is a twelve-step program for cocaine abusers modeled after Alcoholics Anonymous (AA). Support groups and group therapy led by a therapist can be helpful because other addicts can share coping and relapse-prevention strategies. The group's support can help patients face devastating changes and life issues. Some experts recommend that patients be cocaine-free for at least two weeks before participating in a group, but other experts argue that a two-week waiting period is unnecessary and counterproductive. Group counseling sessions led by drug counselors who are in recovery themselves are also useful for some people overcoming their addictions. These group counseling sessions differ from group therapy in that the people in a counseling group are constantly changing.

Medications

Many medications—greater than twenty—have been tested but none have been found to reduce the intensity of withdrawal. Dopamine agonists like amantadine and bromocriptine and tricyclic antidepressants such as desipramine have failed in studies to help treat symptoms of cocaine withdrawal or intoxication.

CANNABIS AND RELATED DISORDERS

Definition

Cannabis, more commonly called marijuana, refers to the several varieties of *Cannabis sativa,* or Indian hemp plant, that contains the psychoactive drug delta-9-tetrahydrocannabinol (THC). Cannabis-related disorders refer to problems associated with the use of substances derived from this plant.

Cannabis intoxication: Cannabis intoxication refers to the occurrence of problematic behaviors or psychological changes that develop during, or shortly after, cannabis use. Intoxication usually starts with a "high" feeling followed by euphoria, inappropriate laughter, and feelings of grandiosity. Other symptoms include sedation, lethargy, impaired short-term memory, difficulty with motor tasks, impaired judgment, distorted sensory perceptions, and the feeling that time is passing unusually slowly. Sometimes severe anxiety, feelings of depression, or social withdrawal may occur. Along with these symptoms, common signs of cannabis intoxication include reddening of the membranes around the eyes, increased appetite, dry mouth, and increased heart rate.

Treatments

Treatment options for individuals with cannabis-related disorders are identical to those available for people with alcohol and other substance abuse disorders. The goal of treatment is abstinence. Treatment approaches range from inpatient hospitalization, drug and alcohol rehabilitation facilities, and various outpatient programs. Twelve-step programs such as Narcotics Anonymous are also treatment options. For heavy users suffering from withdrawal symptoms, treatment with anti-anxiety and/or antidepressant medication may assist in the treatment process.

CAFFEINE–RELATED DISORDER

Definition

Caffeine is a white, bitter crystalline alkaloid derived from coffee or tea. It belongs to a class of compounds called xanthines, its chemical formula being 1, 3, 7-trimethylxanthine. Caffeine is classified together with cocaine and amphatamines as an analeptic, or central nervous system stimulant. Coffee is the most abundant source of caffeine, although caffeine is also found in tea, cocoa, and cola beverages as well as in over-the-counter and prescription medications for pain relief.

Caffeine-related disorders are often unrecognized for a number of reasons:
- Caffeine has a "low profile" as a drug of abuse. Consumption of drinks containing caffeine is unregulated by law and is nearly universal in the United States; one well-known textbook of pharmacology refers to caffeine as "the most widely used psychoactive drug in the world." In many countries, coffee

is a social lubricant as well as a stimulant; the "coffee break" is a common office ritual, and many people find it difficult to imagine eating a meal in a fine restaurant without having coffee at some point during the meal. It is estimated that 10–12 billion pounds of coffee are consumed worldwide each year.
- People often underestimate the amount of caffeine they consume on a daily basis because they think of caffeine only in connection with coffee as a beverage. Tea, cocoa, and some types of soft drink, including root beer and orange soda as well as cola beverages, also contain significant amounts of caffeine. In one British case study, a teenager who was hospitalized with muscle weakness, nausea, vomiting, diarrhea, and weight loss was found to suffer from caffeine intoxication caused by drinking 8 liters (about 2 gallons) of cola on a daily basis for the previous two years. She had been consuming over a gram of caffeine per day. Chocolate bars and coffee-flavored yogurt or ice cream are additional sources of measurable amounts of caffeine.
- Caffeine has some legitimate medical uses in athletic training and in the relief of tension-type headaches. It is available in over-the-counter (OTC) preparations containing aspirin or acetaminophen for pain relief as well as in such OTC stimulants as NoDoz and Vivarin.
- Caffeine is less likely to produce the same degree of physical or psychological dependence as other drugs of abuse. Few coffee or tea drinkers report loss of control over caffeine intake, or significant difficulty in reducing or stopping consumption of beverages and food items containing caffeine.
- The symptoms of caffeine intoxication are easy to confuse with those of an anxiety disorder.

Description

Pharmacological Aspects of Caffeine

An outline of the effects of caffeine on the central nervous system (CNS) and other organ systems of the body may be helpful in understanding its potential for physical dependence. When a person drinks a beverage containing caffeine (or eats coffee-flavored ice cream), the caffeine is absorbed from the digestive tract without being broken down. It is rapidly distributed throughout the tissues of the body by means of the bloodstream. If a pregnant woman drinks a cup of coffee or tea, the caffeine in the drink will cross the placental barrier and enter the baby's bloodstream.

When the caffeine reaches the brain, it increases the secretion of norepinephrine, a neurotransmitter that is associated with the so-called fight or flight stress response. The rise in norepinephrine levels and the increased activity of the neurons, or nerve cells, in many other areas of the brain helps to explain why the symptoms of caffeine intoxication resemble the symptoms of a panic attack.

The effects of caffeine are thought to occur as a result of competitive antagonism at adenosine receptors. Adenosine is a water-soluble compound of adenine and

ribose; it functions to modulate the activities of nerve cells and produces a mild sedative effect when it activates certain types of adenosine receptors. Caffeine competes with adenosine to bind at these receptors and counteracts the sedative effects of the adenosine. If the person stops drinking coffee, the adenosine has no competition for activating its usual receptors and may produce a sedative effect that is experienced as fatigue or drowsiness.

Caffeine can produce a range of physical symptoms following ingestion of as little as 100 mg, although amounts of 250 mg or higher are usually needed to produce symptoms that meet the criteria of caffeine intoxication.

Symptoms

The symptoms of caffeine intoxication include: Restlessness, nervousness, excitement, insomnia, flushed face, diuresis (increased urinary output), gastrointestinal disturbance, muscle twitching, talking or thinking in a rambling manner, tachycardia (speeded-up heartbeat) or disturbances of heart rhythm, periods of inexhaustibility, psychomotor agitation.

People have reported ringing in the ears or seeing flashes of light at doses of caffeine above 250 mg. Profuse sweating and diarrhea have also been reported. Doses of caffeine higher than 10 g may produce respiratory failure, fits and eventually death.

Side Effects and Complications

High short-term consumption of caffeine can produce or worsen gastrointestinal problems, occasionally leading to peptic ulcers or hematemesis (vomiting blood).

In addition to the symptoms produced by high short-term doses, long-term consumption of caffeine has been associated with fertility problems and with bone loss in women leading to osteoporosis in old age. Some studies have found that pregnant women who consume more than 150 mg per day of caffeine have an increased risk of miscarriage and low birth weight babies, but the findings are complicated by the fact that most women who drink large amounts of coffee during pregnancy are also heavy smokers. Some researchers believe that long-term consumption of caffeine is implicated in cardiovascular diseases, but acknowledge that further research is required.

On the other hand, moderate doses of caffeine improve athletic performance as well as alertness. Caffeine in small doses can relieve tension headaches, and one study found that a combination of ibuprofen and caffeine was more effective in relieving tension headaches than either ibuprofen alone or a placebo. Coffee consumption also appears to lower the risk of alcoholic and nonalcoholic cirrhosis of the liver.

Treatments

Treatment of caffeine-related disorders involves lowering consumption levels or abstaining from beverages containing caffeine. Some people experience

mild withdrawal symptoms that include headaches, irritability, and occasionally nausea, but these usually resolve quickly.

Caffeine consumption has the advantage of having relatively weak (compared to alcohol or cigarettes) social reinforcement, in the sense that one can easily choose a noncaffeinated or decaffeinated beverage in a restaurant or at a party without attracting comment. Thus, physical dependence on caffeine is less complicated by the social factors that reinforce nicotine and other drug habits.

AMPHETAMINES AND RELATED DISORDER

Definition

Amphetamines are a group of powerful and highly addictive substances that dramatically affect the central nervous system. They induce a feeling of well-being and improve alertness, attention, and performance on various cognitive and motor tasks. Closely related are the socalled "designer amphetamines," the most well known of which is the "club drug" MDMA, best known as "ecstasy." Finally, some over-the-counter drugs used as appetite suppressant also have amphetamine-like action.

Description

These include dextroamphetamine (Dexedrine), methamphetamine (Desoxyn), and methylphenidate (Ritalin). These Schedule II stimulants, known to be highly addictive, require a triplicate prescription that cannot be refilled. Amphetamines are also known as sympathomimetics, stimulants, and psychostimulants. Methamphetamine, the most common illegally produced amphetamine, goes by the street name of "speed," "meth," and "chalk". When it is smoked, it is called "ice," "crystal," "crank," and "glass". Methamphetamine is a white, odorless, bitter-tasting crystalline powder that dissolves in water or alcohol.

Amphetamines were initially produced for medical use, and were first used in nasal decongestants and bronchial inhalers. Early in the 1900s, they were also used to treat several medical and psychiatric conditions, including narolepsy (a rare condition in which an individuals falls asleep at dangerous and inappropriate moments and cannot maintain normal alertness), attention-deficit disorders, obesity and depression. They are still used to treat these disorders today.

Amphetamine intoxication refers to serious behavioral or psychological changes that develop during, or shortly after, use of amphetamine. Intoxication begins with a "high" feeling, followed by euphoria, enhanced energy, talkativeness, hyperactivity, restlessness, hypervigilance indicated by an individual's extreme sensitivity, and closely observant of everything in the environment). Other symptoms are anxiety, tension, repetitive behavior, anger, fighting, and impaired judgment. With chronic intoxication, there may be fatigue or sadness and withdrawal from others. Other signs and symptoms of intoxication are increased heartrate, dilation of the pupils, elevated or lowered blood pressure, perspiration

or chills, nausea or vomiting, weight loss, cardiac irregularities and, eventually, confusion, seizures, coma, or death.

During amphetamine withdrawal, intense symptoms of depression are typical. Additional diagnostic symptoms are fatigue, vivid and unpleasant dreams, insomnia or sleeping too much, increased appetite, and agitation.

Treatments

No specific medications are known to exist that are helpful for treating amphetamine dependence. On occasion, antidepressant medications can help combat the depressive symptoms frequently experienced by newly abstinent amphetamine users.

Overdoses of amphetamines are treated in established ways in emergency rooms. Because hyperthermia (elevated body temperature), and convulsions are common, emergency room treatment focuses on reducing body temperature and administering anticonvulsant medications.

Acute methamphetamine intoxication is often handled by observation in a safe, quiet environment. When extreme anxiety or panic is part of the reaction, treatment with anti-anxiety medications may be helpful. In cases of methamphetamine-induced psychoses, short-term use of antipsychotic medications is usually successful.

INHALANTS USE DISORDER

Definition

The inhalants are a class of drugs that include a broad range of chemicals found in hundreds of different products, many of which are readily available to the general population. These chemicals include volatile solvents (liquids that vaporize at room temperature) and aerosols (sprays that contain solvents and propellants). Examples include glue, gasoline, paint thinner, hair spray, lighter fluid, spray paint, nail polish remover, correction fluid, rubber cement, felt-tip marker fluids, vegetable sprays, and certain cleaners. The inhalants share a common route of administration— that is, they are all drawn into the body by breathing. They are usually taken either by breathing in the vapors directly from a container (known as "sniffing"); by inhaling fumes from substances placed in a bag (known as "bagging"); or by inhaling the substance from a cloth soaked in it (known as "huffing"). Inhalants take effect very quickly because they get into the bloodstream rapidly via the lungs. The "high" from inhalants is usually brief, so that users often take inhalants repeatedly over several hours. This pattern of use can be dangerous, leading to unconsciousness or even death.

Inhalant intoxication

Intoxication from inhalants occurs rapidly (usually within five minutes) and lasts for a short period of time (from 5 to 30 minutes). Inhalants typically have a depressant effect on the central nervous system, similar to the effects of alcohol;

and produce feelings of euphoria (feeling good), excitement, dizziness, and slurred speech. In addition, persons intoxicated by inhalants may feel as if they are floating, or feel a sense of increased power. Severe intoxication from inhalants can cause coma or even death.

Treatments

Chronic inhalant users are difficult to treat because they often have many serious personal and social problems. They also have difficulty staying away from inhalants; relapse rates are high. Treatment usually takes a long-time and involves enlisting the support of the person's family; changing the friendship network if the individual uses with others; teaching coping skills; and increasing self-esteem.

HALLUCINOGENS AND RELATED DISORDER

Hallucinogens are a chemically diverse group of drugs that cause changes in a person's thought processes, perceptions of the physical world, and sense of time passing. Hallucinogens can be found naturally in some plants, and can be synthesized in the laboratory. Most hallucinogens are abused as recreational drugs. Hallucinogens are also called psychedelic drugs.

Description

Most hallucinogens are synthesized in illegal laboratories for delivery as street drugs. The best known hallucinogens are lysergic acid diethylamide (LSD), mescaline, psilocybin, and MDMA (ecstasy). Phencyclidine (PCP, angel dust) can produce hallucinations, as can amphetamines and marijuana, but these drugs are not considered classic hallucinogens and are discussed under separate entries. In addition, new designer drugs that are chemical variants of classic hallucinogens are apt to appear on the street at any time.

Lysergic Acid Diethylamide (LSD)

LSD is the best known and most potent of the hallucinogens. LSD was first synthesized by Alfred Hoffman for a pharmaceutical company in Germany in 1938 while searching for a headache remedy. Hoffman discovered the hallucinogenic properties of LSD accidentally in 1943. The drug became popular with hippies in the mid-1960s when its sense-altering properties were reputed to offer a window into enhanced creativity and self-awareness. LSD also occurs naturally in morning glory seeds.

Pure LSD is a white, odorless, crystalline powder that dissolves easily in water, although contaminants can cause it to range in color from yellow to dark brown. LSD was listed as a schedule I drug under the Controlled Substance Act of 1970, meaning that it has no medical or legal uses and has a high potential for abuse. LSD is not easy to manufacture in a home laboratory, and some of its ingredients are controlled substances that are difficult to obtain. However, LSD is very potent, and a small amount can produce a large number of doses.

On the street, LSD is sold in several forms. Microdots are tiny pills smaller than a pinhead. Windowpane is liquid LSD applied to thin squares of gelatin. Liquid LSD can also be sprayed on sugar cubes. The most common street form of the drug is liquid LSD sprayed onto blotter paper and dried. The paper, often printed with colorful or psychedelic pictures, is divided into tiny squares, each square being one dose. Liquid LSD can also be sprayed on the back of a postage stamp and licked off. Street names for the drug include acid, yellow sunshine, windowpane, doses, trips, and boomers.

Mescaline

Mescaline is a naturally occurring plant hallucinogen. Its primary source is the cactus *Lophophora williamsii*. This cactus is native to the South-Western United States and Mexico. The light blue-green plant is spineless and has a crown called a peyote button. This button contains mescaline and can be eaten or made into a bitter tea. Mescaline is also the active ingredient of at least ten other cacti of the genus *Trichocereus* that are native to parts of South America.

Psilocybin

Psilocybin is the active ingredient in what are known on the street as magic mushrooms, shrooms, mushies, or Mexican mushrooms. There are several species of mushrooms that contain psilocybin, including *Psilocybe mexicana, P. muscorumi,* and *Stropharia cubensis*. These mushrooms grow in most moderate, moist climates.

MDMA

MDMA, short for 3, 4-methylenedioxymethamphetamine, and better known as ecstasy, TXC, E, X, or Adam, has become an increasingly popular club drug since the 1980s. MDMA was first synthesized in 1912 by a German pharmaceutical company looking for a new compound that would stop bleeding. The company patented the drug, but never did anything with it. A closely related drug, methylenedioxyamphetimine or MDA, was tested by a pharmaceutical company as an appetite suppressant in the 1950s, but its use was discontinued when it was discovered to have hallucinogenic properties. In the 1960s, MDA was a popular drug of abuse in some large cities such as San Francisco.

Causes and Symptoms

Psychological symptoms of hallucinogen intoxication include:
- Distortion of sight, sound, and touch
- Confusion of the senses—sounds are "seen" or vision is "heard"
- Disorientation in time and space
- Delusions of physical invulnerability (especially with LSD)
- Paranoia
- Unreliable judgment and increased risk taking
- Anxiety attacks

- Flashbacks after the drug has been cleared from the body
- Blissful calm or mellowness
- Reduced inhibitions
- Increased empathy (MDMA)
- Elation or euphoria
- Impaired concentration and motivation
- Long-term memory loss
- Personality changes, especially if there is a latent psychiatric disorder
- Psychological drug dependence.

Physical Symptoms

Although the primary effects of hallucinogens are on perceptions, some physical effects do occur. Physical symptoms include: Increased blood pressure, increased heart rate, nausea and vomiting (especially with psilocybin and mescaline), blurred vision which can last after the drug has worn off, poor coordination, enlarged pupils, sweating, diarrhea (plant hallucinogens), restlessness, muscle cramping (especially clenched jaws with MDMA), dehydration (MDMA) and serious increase in body temperature leading to seizures (MDMA).

Treatments

Acute treatment is aimed at preventing the patient from harming himself or anyone else. Since most people experiencing hallucinogen intoxication remain in touch with reality, "talking down" or offering reassurance and support that emphasizes that the bad trip, anxiety, panic attack, or paranoia will pass as the drug wears off is often helpful. Patients are kept in a calm, pleasant, but lighted environment, and are encouraged to move around while being helped to remain oriented to reality. Occasionally, drugs such as lorazepam are given for anxiety. Complications in treatment occur when the hallucinogen has been contaminated with other street drugs or chemicals. The greatest life-threatening risk is associated with MDMA. Users may develop dangerously high body temperatures. Reducing the patient's temperature is an essential acute treatment.

Treatment for long-term effects of hallucinogen use involve long-term psychotherapy after drug use has stopped. Many people find 12-step programs or group support helpful. In addition, underlying psychiatric disorders must be addressed.

Chapter 8

Psychophysiological Disorders

ANOREXIA NERVOSA

Definition

Anorexia nervosa is an eating disorder characterized by following features:
- Most often occur in females than males
- Common age of onset in adolescence (13–19 years)
- Intense fear of becoming obese
- Body image disturbance
- Refusal to maintain above a minimum normal body weight for age, sex, height
- Significant loss of weight—usually more than 25% of the original body weight or BMI below 17.5
- No medical illness
- Absence psychiatric illness
- Primary or secondary amenorrhea
- Strict dietary restrictions
- Poor sexual adjustment and fear of pregnancy (unable to accept the 'female role').

Comorbidity

Depressive symptoms and obsessive compulsive personality traits and about 50% of anorectics have bulimic episodes with binge eating.

Differential Diagnosis

Medical illness—hypopituitarism, tuberculosis, depressive episodes.

Treatment

- Short-term management—to ensure weight gain and correct nutritional deficiencies
- Long-term treatment aimed at maintaining a normal weight achieved through a short-term management.

Treatment modalities include:
- Behavior therapy—based on positive reinforcement and sometimes negative reinforcements.
- Individual psychotherapy
- Hospitalization—with adequate nursing care

- Pharmacotherapy with CPZ, FXT, AMT, clomipramine and cyproheptadine (8 to 32 mg)
- Group therapy and family therapy

Prognosis

Prognosis is better in:
- Younger age of onset
- Less number of hospitalizations
- No bulimic episodes.

BULIMIA NERVOSA

Definition

Bulimia nervosa is an eating disorder characterized by following clinical features:
- Commonly in early teens and adolescents
- There is intense fear of becoming obese
- Recurrent binge eating large quantities of food
- Feeling of lack of control over eating during binges
- Self-induced purging
- Vomiting, using laxatives, diuretics, fasting or excessive exercise
- Self-evaluation unduly influenced by body shape and weight
- Bingeing and purging are not accompanied by anorexia nervosa.

Treatment

- Behavior therapy
- Based on positive and negative reinforcements
- Individual psychotherapy
- Drugs as adjuncts—imipramine, FXT
- Group therapy and family therapy.

OTHER EATING DISORDERS

Rumination Syndrome

Rumination syndrome is characterized by the repeated painless regurgitation of food following a meal which is then either re-chewed, re-swallowed or discarded. It is an under-diagnosed disorder possibly due to the fact that most physicians do not recognize the symptoms of the disorder. While often diagnosed in infants and developmently individuals it also occurs in adults of normal intelligence.

Food Maintenance Syndrome

Food maintenance syndrome is characterized by a set of aberrant eating behaviors of children in foster care it is "a pattern of excessive eating and food acquisition and maintenance behaviors without concurrent obesity", it resembles "the behavioral correlates of Hyperphagic Short Stature".

Diabulimia

Diabulimia is the term given to the unhealthy practice by which individuals who have type 1 diabetes try to lose weight by depriving themselves of insulin.

Binge Eating Disorder

Binge eating disorder is the most common of all eating disorders, affecting an estimated 2 to 5% of adults. Binge eating disorder involves more than occasional overeating, but rather frequent episodes of bingeing on unusually large amounts of food. Despite feeling ashamed and disgusted, people with binge eating disorder feel an overwhelming compulsion to continue bingeing well beyond the point of fullness.

Warning Signs of Binge Eating Disorder

Because they feel a great deal of shame and powerlessness, individuals with binge eating disorder may go to great lengths to hide their disorder. Even close friends and family members may not realize the individual is suffering so profoundly.

If you are concerned, keep a watchful eye for these symptoms of binge eating disorder:
- Frequently consuming abnormally large amounts of food
- Eating rapidly and until uncomfortably full
- Eating alone or hiding food
- Feeling numb or "out of body" when bingeing
- Feelings of shame, guilt, depression or self-hatred.

Dangers of Binge Eating

Binge eating disorder often leads to obesity, which is responsible for as many as 300,000 deaths per year. The disorder often occurs alongside other conditions, such as substance abuse and psychiatric disorders, such as depression, anxiety disorders and personality disorders.

Some of the medical consequences of binge eating disorder include:
- Heart disease
- Cancer
- Diabetes
- High blood pressure and cholesterol.

Causes

While the causes of bulimia are not fully understood, there is a clear association between binge eating disorder and depression and other mental health disorders. Most likely, there is a genetic component to binge eating disorder. People with the illness often have a history of dieting, weight gain and eating to cope with feelings of anger, boredom, sadness and other painful emotions.

Treatment

Like other eating disorders, binge eating disorder is complex and requires comprehensive treatment to address the underlying emotional and psychological issues as well as any medical complications. Whether an individual is normal weight, overweight or obese, they can benefit from binge eating disorder treatment. Treatment for binge eating disorder may include:
- Cognitive-behavioral therapy
- Dialectical behavior therapy
- Medication
- Family and group therapy
- Weight management and menu planning

In some cases, a stay in a residential eating disorder treatment program offers the best opportunity for lasting recovery. Staffed by eating disorder specialists, these programs take a comprehensive and holistic approach to treating eating disorders before initiating a weight loss plan.

Compulsive Overeating

Compulsive eating, sometimes referred to as binge eating disorder or food addiction, is not its own classification of eating disorder, but like anorexia and bulimia, points to unhealthy behaviors and thought patterns around food and weight.

Causes

Compulsive overeating is caused by a number of factors:
- Family history
- Brain chemistry/metabolism
- Stress
- Trauma
- Emotional or psychological issues.

Symptoms

Compulsive eaters lose control around food and may use food to cope with difficult emotions. They feel compelled to eat even when they are uncomfortably full, sometimes eating very quickly, when they are alone or non-stop throughout the day. If unable to eat the high-fat, high-calorie foods they crave, compulsive overeaters may experience withdrawal-like symptoms.

After overeating, the individual typically feels ashamed and disgusted, which only makes them turn to food once again for comfort.

Treatment

Even though people who compulsively overeat desperately want to stop, their mental state prevents them from doing so. In some cases, the only way to effectively curb compulsive overeating is with professional eating disorder treatment.

In a safe, supportive setting, people who compulsively overeat can get to the source of their eating disorder behaviors and begin to develop healthier habits.

Pica

Pica is an eating disorder characterized by a pattern of eating non-food items such as:
- Dirt or clay
- Ice
- Glue
- Leaves
- Insects
- Paint
- Sand
- Animal waste.

Pica affects children more often than adults, with 10 to 32% of kids ages 1 to 6 displaying these behaviors. Pregnant women are also at greater risk of developing pica.

Causes

Pica may be caused by nutritional deficiencies (such as a lack of iron or zinc) or malnourishment, though scientists are still uncertain of the exact cause. Other possible causes include:
- Developmental delay
- Poverty
- Emotional deprivation or neglect
- Anemia.

The Effects of Pica

Pica should never be ignored. Ingesting materials that were not intended as food can lead to serious medical issues such as:
- Infections
- Lead poisoning
- Intestinal obstruction or perforation.

Treatment

While some people struggle with pica for several months and then stop showing signs of the disorder, others struggle well into adolescence and adulthood and require treatment to overcome this dangerous eating behavior. Treatment for pica typically includes:
- Medical assessments and care
- Therapy
- Medication
- Mild aversion therapy and positive reinforcement.

Obesity

Obesity has become commonplace in our culture, yet it destroys the lives of hundreds of thousands of people each year.

Obesity is defined as:
- Being more than 20% over your ideal body weight (which is based on age, gender and activity level)
- Having more than 30% body fat for women and more than 25% body fat for men.

Causes

While the cause of obesity is simple—more calories consumed than burnt—the root of the disease is much more complex. Obesity can be caused by:
- Genetics
- Overeating
- Consuming too many high-fat, high-calorie foods
- Sedentary lifestyle
- Social and cultural expectations
- Emotional or psychological issues.

Effects of Being Obese

Obesity is responsible for as many as 300,000 deaths each year, according to the Centers for Disease Control and Prevention. Obese individuals are at increased risk for a number of complications, including: Heart disease, stroke, diabetes, certain types of cancer, high blood pressure and cholesterol, depression, complications in pregnancy and eating disorders.

Treatment

Obese individuals often feel a profound sense of shame, loss and isolation. If you are struggling with overweight or obesity, know that you are not alone and your quality of life can be dramatically improved. By learning new skills, adopting new lifestyle habits and engaging in therapy to address any underlying emotional issues, obesity treatment can save lives.

SOMATIZATION DISORDER

The most common characteristic of the somatoform disorder is the appearance of physical symptoms or complaints for which they have no organic basis. Such dysfunctional symptoms tend to range from sensory or motor disability, hypersensitivity to pain. Four major somatoform disorders exist: Conversion disorder (also known as hysteria), hypochondriasis, somatization disorder, and somatoform pain disorder. Somatization disorder is also known as Briquet's Syndrome.

Starting before age 30, the patient has had many physical complaints occurring over several years and has sought treatment for these symptoms, or they have

materially impaired social, work or personal functioning. The patient has at some time experienced a total of at least 8 symptoms from the following list for which the symptoms need not be concurrent.

- **Pain Symptoms** (4 or more) related to different sites, such as head, abdomen, back, joints, extremities, chest or rectum, or related to body functions such as menstruation, sexual intercourse or urination.
- **Gastrointestinal Symptoms** (2 or more, excluding pain) such as nausea, bloating, vomiting (not during pregnancy), diarrhea, intolerance of several foods.
- **Sexual Symptoms** (at least 1, excluding pain) including indifference to sex, difficulties with erection or ejaculation, irregular menses, excessive menstrual bleeding or vomiting throughout all nine months of pregnancy.
- **Pseudoneurological Symptoms** (at least 1) including impaired balance or coordination, weak or paralyzed muscles, lump in throat or trouble swallowing, loss of voice, retention of urine, hallucinations, numbness (to touch or pain), double vision, blindness, deafness, seizures, amnesia or other dissociative symptoms, loss of consciousness (other than with fainting). None of these is limited to pain.

For each of the above symptoms, one of these conditions must be met:
- Physical or laboratory investigation determines that the symptom cannot be fully explained by a general medical condition or by substance use, including medications and drugs of abuse, or
- If the patient does have a general medical condition, the impairment or complaints exceed what you would expect, based on history, laboratory findings or physical examination.
- The patient does not consciously feign the symptoms for material gain (malingering) or to occupy the sick role (factitious disorder).

Symptoms

Vomiting, abdominal pain, nausea, bloating, diarrhea, pain in the arms or legs, back pain, joint pain, pain during urination, headaches, shortness of breath, palpitations, chest pain, dizziness, amnesia, difficulty swallowing, vision changes, paralysis or muscle weakness, sexual apathy, pain during intercourse, impotence, painful menstruation, irregular menses, excessive menstrual bleeding, discussion of other aspects of life may cause anxiety.

Note: A variety of symptoms may be present at any given time.

Associated Features

Many somatic complaints and long, complicated medical histories. Psychological distress and interpersonal problems are prominent. Medical histories are often circumstantial, vague, imprecise, inconsistent and disorganized.

Causes

The cause is not specific but symptoms begin or worsen after losses (for example, job, close relative, or friend). A greater intensity of symptoms often occurs with stress.

Treatment

The goal of treatment is to help the person learn to control the symptoms.

A supportive relationship with a sympathetic health care provider is the most important aspect of treatment. Regularly scheduled appointments should be maintained to review symptoms and the person's coping mechanisms.

Acknowledgment and explanation of test results should occur. It is not helpful to tell the people with this disorder that their symptoms are imaginary. People with a somatization disorder rarely acknowledge that their illness has a psychological component and will usually reject psychiatric treatment.

SLEEP DISORDERS

Definition

Sleep can be defined as a normal state of altered consciousness during which the body rests; it is characterized by decreased responsiveness to the environment, and a person can be aroused from it by external stimuli.

Chronobiology

Chronobiology refers to the study of biologic changes as they occur in relation to time. The *sleep wake cycle* is one of the circadian rhythms of the body. *Circadian rhythms* follow an approximate 24 hours cycle through a complex process linked to light and dark. The effect of illness and hospitalization may disrupt these rhythms, particularly in older persons. *Ultradian cycles* are circadian rhythms of less than 24 hours. The recurrent pattern of sleep stages, repeating approximately 90 minutes in adults, is an example. *Chronopharmacology* refers to the study of how biorhythms affect the absorption, metabolism, and excretion of drugs. For example, the blood level achieved by a continuous infusion of heparin varies throughout the day.

Stages of Sleep

Non-rapid eye movement (NREM) sleep is characterized as follows:
Stage 1:
- Includes lightest level of sleep
- Stage lasts a few minutes
- Decreased physiological activity begins with gradual fall in vital signs and metabolism
- Sensory stimuli such as noise, easily arouse sleeper
- If awakened, person feels as though daydreaming has occurred.

Stage 2:
- Includes period of sound sleep
- Relaxation progresses
- Arousal is still relatively easy
- Stage lasts 10–20 minutes
- Body functions continue to slow.

The brain waves are frequently mixed and low voltage in pattern, with bursts of activity called sleep spindles and large amplitude waves called K complexes.

Stage 3:
- It involves initial stages of deep sleep
- Sleeper is difficult to arouse and rarely moves
- Oxygen consumption
- Muscles are completely relaxed
- Vital signs decline, but remain regular
- Stage lasts 15–30 minutes.

Stage 4:
- It is deepest stage of sleep
- It is very difficult to arouse sleeper
- If sleep loss has occurred, sleeper will spend considerable portion of night in this stage
- Vital signs are significantly lower than during waking hours
- Stage lasts approximately 15–30 minutes
- Sleep walking and enuresis sometimes occur
- Stage 3 and 4 known as slow wave sleep, named for the characteristic high voltage and low-frequency delta waves.

Rapid eye movement (REM) sleep:
- Vivid, full-color dreaming occurs
- Stage usually begins about 90 minutes after sleep has begun
- Stage typified by autonomic responses of rapidly moving eyes, fluctuating heart and respiratory rates, and increased or fluctuating blood pressure
- Loss of skeletal muscle tone occurs
- Gastric secretion increase
- It is very difficult to arouse sleeper
- Duration of REM sleep increases with each cycle and averages 20 minutes
- Stage is characterized by low voltage, random fast waves, as in stage 1 NREM.

Sleep Pattern Disturbance

Sleep pattern disturbance is defined as a disruption of sleep time that causes discomfort or interferes with a desired life cycle. A sleep pattern disturbance may be related to one of more than 80 sleep disorders identified in the international classification of sleep disorders, a partial list of which is given below:

I. Dyssomnias

The Dyssomnias include sleep disorders characterized by difficulty in initiating or maintaining sleep (insomnia) or by excessive sleepiness. These disorders

may arise predominantly from within the body (intrinsic), from external sources (extrinsic), or from disruption of circadian rhythm.

A. Intrinsic Sleep Disorders

1. Insomnia

It is the persistent difficulty in initiating or maintaining sleep. The difficulty does not respond readily to improved sleep habits or removal of precipitating factors. ***Idiopathic insomnia*** is a rare disorder characterized by a lifelong history of inability to obtain adequate sleep. Its cause is thought to be an abnormality in the neurologic control of sleep. ***Psychophysiologic insomnia*** is more common and is characterized by learned sleep preventing associations and heightened physiologic response to stress. It can be confirmed by polysomnographic recording, which usually shows the same pattern of long sleep latency or fragmentation that the client describes. The total sleep time is often within normal range but is felt to be inadequate. They will fall asleep unintentionally in low stimulus situations, such as watching TV, but feel increased arousal when they go to bed. It is difficult to get sleep in places, other than their usual bedroom.

Management of insomnia is complex. Sleep should be restricted by curtailing time bed to the minimum believed necessary with a consistent rising time. Relaxation exercises can be helpful, but they should initially be practiced at times other than bedtime, so that by the time they are introduced at bedtime, they are effective. Referral to a sleep specialist or mental health professional who can work with the client over a period of time should be considered.

2. Narcolepsy

Narcolepsy is one of the disorders characterized by excessive daytime sleepiness. The client also experiences disturbed nocturnal sleep and repeated episodes of almost irresistible daytime drowsiness followed by brief periods of sleep, especially when engaged in monotonous activities. Many narcoleptic clients also experience ***cataplexy,*** a sudden loss of muscle tone at times of unexpected emotion (e.g. fright). Malfunctioning of the mechanism controlling REM sleep leads to ***sleep paralysis*** for one to several minutes, and ***hypnagogic hallucinations***, i.e. hallucinatory experiences that occur at sleep onset or awakening.

On polysomnography, the most characteristic finding is sleep onset REM periods. Narcolepsy is genetically related condition with autosomal dominance in some cases. The effects of disease on lifestyle are significant—many clients reporting episodes of having fallen asleep at work, while driving, or both.

Medical management consists of low doses of stimulants to improve alertness and tricyclic antidepressants to control cataplexy. It is important that they maintain a regular schedule with adequate nocturnal sleep. Recommend regular naps at times when clients are prone to increased sleepiness. Safety is the major issue in these clients.

3. Sleep apnea syndrome

Sleep apnea is characterized by cessation of breathing for 10 seconds or longer occuring at least 5 times/hour. Sleep apnea can be classified as obstructive and central nervous system apnea. A combination of the two may be seen.

Obstructive sleep apnea syndrome: In obstructive sleep apnea syndrome, respiratory efforts of the diaphragm and intercostals muscles are apparent but ineffective against a collapsed or obstructed upper airway. Snoring indicates partial obstruction. As hypoxia ensues; the person eventually awakens to breathe. The frequent awakenings impair the normal sleep cycle. Repeated microarousals lead to daytime sleepiness.

Women are less likely than men to develop obstructive sleep apnea syndrome, particularly before menopause. It is common among males who are obese with short, thick necks, and who are heavy snorers. A much smaller percentage progresses to the classic pickwickian syndrome, characterized by obesity, severe sleep apnea, daytime hypercapnea, and cor pulmonale.

The application of continuous positive airway pressure (CPAP) by means of a face mask covering the nose is the treatment of choice for clients with moderate to severe obstructive sleep apnea syndrome. The CPAP device provides room air under increased pressure, essentially providing a pressure splint to keep the upper airway open. It should be turned on whenever the client is ready to go to sleep and should be maintained throughout the sleep period. Clients may experience nasal congestion, air leak, pressure marks on the face, or pressure intolerance. People who use CPAP regularly should bring their units to the hospital with them. These clients need to be monitored when recovering from anesthesia, and when receiving narcotics because they are at risk for developing ineffective breathing patterns.

Uvulopalatopharyngoplasty is a common surgical procedure for reducing snoring. Resecting the uvula, the posterior part of the soft palate, tonsils and any excessive pharyngeal tissue, can reduce the propensity to obstruction. Tracheostomy may be required in severe obstructive sleep apnea syndrome.

Central sleep apnea syndrome: It is characterized by apneic periods during which no apparent respiratory effort occurs. It may be seen in stroke and brain stem involvement, but it is most commonly mixed with obstructive sleep apnea syndrome. Cheyne-Stokes respirations are common, and CPAP is the usual treatment.

4. Periodic limb movement disorder

It may also contribute to daytime sleepiness and frequent nocturnal wakening. Originally described as nocturnal myoclonus, it is characterized by periodic episodes of repetitive, stereotypic leg movements that occur during sleep, causing partial arousals. It is common in the elderly population. Clonazepam, a benzodiazepine, or baclofen, a skeletal muscle relaxant, may be ordered to diminish the magnitude of the movement and frequency of arousals. For some clients the use of transcutaneous electrical nerve stimulation (TENS) before sleep has been helpful.

5. Restless leg syndrome
Restless leg syndrome involves anything "crawling", itching or tingling sensations of the leg while at rest and causes an almost irresistible urge to move. The syndrome is often most severe before sleep onset. Clients always have periodic limb movements during sleep. Treatment is similar to that of periodic limb movement disorder.

B. Extrinsic Sleep Disorders

It encompasses a range of factors, from environmentally to chemically induced. Some environmental factors temporarily present during hospitalization.

Circadian rhythm sleep disorders
In the general population, the circadian rhythm sleep disorders, such as ***time zone change syndrome*** and ***shift work sleep disorder*** are not uncommon. Elderly and chronically ill clients who live alone may be vulnerable to irregular sleep-wake patterns. In this disorder, prolonged ignoring or absence of external cues to time, such as regular meal timings, work periods and daylight leads to erratic periods of sleeping and wakefulness. Internal circadian cues may also be damped as a result of ageing or diffuse brain disease.

Management includes maintenance of regular schedule and exposure to natural sunlight. Light therapy is being used to facilitate adjustments in circadian rhythms. The usual dosage is about 5000 lux-hours, which may be taken as 2500 lux for 2 hours, 5000 lux for 1 hour, or 10,000 lux for 30 minutes. It should begin only under the guidance of a physician. Side effects include eyestrain, headache and irritability. Presence of retinopathy, glaucoma or cataract is a contraindication.

II. Parasomnias

The Parasomnias are disorders that occur during sleep but that usually do not produce insomnia or excessive sleepiness. It may be due to partial arousal or abnormalities in sleep-wake transition.

A. Arousal Disorders

Partial arousal occur during slow-wave sleep. ***Sleepwalking***, also known as ***somnambulism***, may include semi-purposeful behavior, such as dressing. However, the behavior may be lacking in coordination and appropriateness, such as voiding in the closet. The occurrence of sleep walking in adults is associated with anxiety. ***Sleep terrors*** are sudden arousals from slow wave sleep accompanied by screaming, tachycardia, tachypnea, diaphoresis, and other manifestations of fear. If awakened, the person is often disoriented and has little recall of the nature of the dream image. Sleep terrors usually occurs in young children.

B. Sleep-wake Transition Disorders

Sleep-wake transition disorders are common in the general population. ***Sleep starts*** refers to the sudden jerking movement of the legs that often occurs as a

person is falling asleep. Nocturnal leg cramps also common. The frequency and intensity may be greater with high caffeine intake, stress, or intense physical activity before going to bed. **Sleep talking** also may occur during times of stress.

C. Parasomnias usually Associated with REM Sleep

Nightmares are frightening dreams that arise in REM sleep and are often vividly recalled on awakening. **Sleep paralysis** is one of the classic signs of narcolepsy, but can occur in isolation. This effect may be an extension of the normal state of low muscle tone during REM sleep.

D. Other Parasomnias

Other Parasomnias are not specifically associated with particular sleep stage. **Sleep bruxism** refers to grinding of the teeth during sleep and may lead to dental damage. **Sleep enuresis**, or bed wetting, may occur in adult in association with other disorders, such as obstructive sleep apnea syndrome. **Primary snoring** is distinguished from obstructive sleep apnea syndrome by its rhythmic nature without episodes of apnea or hypoventilation.

III. Sleep Disorders Associated with Medical or Psychiatric Disorders

A. Neurotransmitter Imbalances

Neurotransmitter imbalances predispose to sleep pattern disturbances. It is more common in case of Parkinson's disease, depression, and Alzheimer's disease. These imbalances may be disease related or drug-induced.

B. Head Injury

Head injury of all degrees of severity affects sleep pattern. For clients in the confused, agitated stage of recovery that results from more severe head injury, use of environmental cues (e.g. light and darkness), regularity of daily schedule, and appropriate daytime exercise and activity can help to restore the sleep-wake cycle.

C. Hormonal Imbalances

Hormonal imbalances also contribute to sleep pattern disorders. Hyperthyroid clients tend to have fragmented, short sleep periods with an excess of slow wave sleep. Hypothyroidism is characterized by excessive sleepiness, and polysomnographic recordings show a reduction in the proportion of slow-wave sleep. Clients with type 1 diabetes mellitus may experience hypoglycemic attacks during the night. Sleep patterns normally vary across the menstrual cycle in response to estrogen and progesterone levels. Women with premenstrual syndrome tend to have less slow-wave sleep throughout the menstrual cycle than their asymptomatic peers. Postmenopausal women are at higher risk for experiencing snoring and obstructive sleep apnea syndrome.

D. Respiratory Disorders

Chronic airway limitations such as asthma and emphysema contribute to difficulty in initiating sleep, frequent arousals with shortness of breath or cough, and chronic fatigue. Some medications such as theophylline preparations may contribute to insomnia.

E. Cardiovascular Disorders

The Cardiovascular diseases such as hypertension, myocardial infarction, and nocturnal angina leads to obstructive sleep apnea, hypoxemia, frequent arousals, increased stage 1 sleep, and reduced total sleep time.

F. Gastrointestinal Disorders

In duodenal ulcer, gastric acid secretion is higher than average and recurrent awakenings with epigastric pain are common, especially in the first 4 hours and antacids needs to be administered. Advice to raise the head of the bed on blocks and to avoid eating within 3 hours of bedtime to avoid gastroesophageal reflux that may lead to esophagitis in severe cases.

G. Other Disorders

Numerous other disorders such as, skin conditions (atopic eczema), fibromyalgia, and seizures seem to have an effect on or an association with sleep.

IV. Hospital Acquired Sleep Disturbances

Clients in the hospital may report various types of sleep disturbances. The etiologic mechanism and intervention may differ from each other.

A. Sleep Onset Difficulty

It is because of the strange environment and the anxieties associated with illness and hospitalization. Environmental control, such as reduction of noise and interruptions, and conservative relaxation measures, such as a back rub should be tried before resorting to a hypnotic agent.

B. Sleep Maintenance Disturbance

It may be associated with substance use or withdrawal from a variety of medications and related substances. Alcohol hastens sleep onset but leads to awakening later in the night. Internal stimuli, such as pain, discomfort, and the urge to void are frequent disturbers of sleep. External stimuli include environmental factors, such as light, noise, temperature, as well as disruptions by other people. Nocturnal stimuli can be reduced by darkening the room, turn lights off, close curtains, reduce noise, adjust temperature by providing bed coverings, spacing necessary care giving activities, and by coordinating the nature and timings of interruptions by other care givers.

C. Early Morning Awakening

It occurs frequently among elderly. Sleep is disturbed in depression and delirium, and is grossly disturbed with frightening dreams, disorientation and restlessness.

D. Sleep Deprivation

The noise level, 24 hours lighting, and frequency of care giver interruptions create sensory overload and sleep deprivation, which is thought to be a major factor contributing to postoperative psychosis.

Assessment and Management

Diagnostic Assessment

- Polysomnography
- Electroencephalogram
- Multiple sleep latency test (MSLT)

MSLT is performed to assess the impairment of daytime alertness. It is performed a day after a standard polysomnogram. The time required for clients to fall asleep when in a relaxed state is evaluated at 2 hours intervals, with each nap limited to 20 minutes. The type of sleep also is assessed.

Chapter 9

Personality Disorders

'Personality Disorder' is a controversial diagnosis, covering a wide range of different attitudes and behaviors and affecting an estimated 10% of the general population. The term is generally used to describe behaviors that do not fit into any other obvious diagnostic category, but where the person nevertheless has difficulty coping with life and where that behavior persistently causes distress to themselves or others. Common problems include having difficulty in sustaining relationships and interpreting social cues. At present there is no consensus as to its causes or treatment.

There are various different types of personality disorders but all of them share the following features:
- Most often the first signs of a personality disorder appear in late childhood or adolescence and continue during adulthood.
- Personality disorders in children or adolescence are sometimes described as conduct disorders. However, most conduct disorders in children do not necessarily lead to personality disorders in adults.
- Someone with a personality disorder holds attitudes and behaves in ways that can cause considerable problems for themselves and others. For example, the way they perceive the world; the way they think; the way they relate to other people; the way they do or do not get upset.
- People diagnosed with personality disorder may be inflexible in that they may have a narrow range of attitudes, behaviors and coping mechanisms.
- These ways of behaving are long standing.

Other key points:
- Most people diagnosed with a personality disorder fit the criteria for at least two different types of personality disorder.
- Most people diagnosed with a personality disorder are not dangerous.
- Dangerousness is most often but not exclusively associated with anti-social or psychopathic disorder.
- People diagnosed as borderline or paranoid personality disorder may be at higher risk of self harm and/or suicide than other people.
- People with personality disorders have multiple needs and vulnerabilities.

TYPES OF PERSONALITY DISORDERS

- Anti-social personality disorder
- Anxious personality disorder

- Dependant personality disorder
- Emotionally unstable personality disorder
- Histrionic personality disorder
- Narcissistic personality disorder
- Obsessive-compulsive personality disorder
- Paranoid personality disorder
- Schizoid personality disorder
- Schizotypal personality disorder.

Anti-Social (Dissocial) Personality Disorder

- Appear to be callous and unconcerned about how their behavior makes other people feel, they do not feel guilt or profit from experience (for instance punishment). On the other hand will tend to blame other people for their problems or to find a way of rationalizing what they have done
- Because of their disregard for social norms, rules and obligations they act in ways that are regarded as unacceptably and grossly irresponsible
- Cannot cope with a long-term relationship, although forming one is not problematic
- Cannot tolerate frustration and are prone to outbursts of aggression and violence.

Anxious (Avoidant) Personality Disorder

- Persistent and pervasive feelings of shyness, insecurity, apprehension and tension leading to restrictions in lifestyle.
- Believing oneself to be unlikeable, undeserving, socially inept, and less important than other people leading to a reluctance to get involved in relationships unless certain of being liked.
- Over-concerned by the fear of being criticized or rejected in social or work situations leading to an avoidance of any activity that involves having to inter-relate with other people.

Dependant Personality Disorder

- Encouraging or allowing others to make important life decisions and a limited ability to make every day decisions unless given excessive reassurance and advice.
- Unwilling to make demands on people, especially those people who play an important part in their life and by doing so becoming compliant and subordinate to other peoples wishes.
- Feelings of helplessness and discomfort when alone and anxiety about being abandoned by loved ones due to fears of being unable to care for themselves.

Emotionally Unstable Personality Disorder

There are two kinds of emotionally unstable personality disorder—'impulsive type' and 'borderline type'. They both share the following characteristics:
- A marked tendency to act impulsively without considering the consequences of these actions, for example engaging in unprotected sex or substance abuse
- An inability to plan ahead, coupled with a lack of self control and outbursts of intense anger, which can lead to violence and other extreme behavior, especially if impulsive acts are challenged or prevented by people around them.

The Impulsive type: Characterized by emotional instability and an inability to control impulses, with episodes of threatening behavior and violence occurring particularly in response to criticism by others.

The Borderline type: Also characterized by emotional instability. In addition, people with this type of personality disorder may experience severe doubts about their self image, aims and sexual preferences which cause upset and distress. It is common to experience a strong and debilitating sense of emptiness and this can lead to self harm and suicide threats. Liable to become involved in intense but unstable relationships which can cause them continual emotional crises, which they will endure to avoid being abandoned.

Histrionic Personality Disorder

- Given to theatricality, self dramatization and exaggerating the expression of emotions
- Suggestible and easily influenced by others or circumstances
- A need to constantly find activities offering excitement and the opportunity to be the center of attention and a longing to be appreciated by other people
- Over concern with physical attractiveness
- A tendency to act or appear in an inappropriately seductive way
- A tendency to be persistently manipulative to achieve what they want and to be easily hurt if obstructed.

Narcissistic Personality Disorder

- Arrogant and self important
- Fantasises about unlimited successes and achievements
- Believes that they are special and can only be understood by other special people
- Constant need for attention and admiration
- Exploits others to achieve own ends
- Lacks empathy is unwilling to recognize or identify with the feelings and needs of others
- Is often envious of others or believes that others are envious of them.

Obsessive-Compulsive (Anankastic) Personality Disorder

- Feelings of excessive doubt and caution compensated by a need to adhere strictly to rules, lists and orders, although paradoxically this perfectionism often interferes with the successful completion of tasks.
- Close relationships and pleasurable activities are difficult to maintain in the face of the need to meet excessive standards of conscientiousness and productivity. This attitude is off putting to other people especially as they expect the same dedication from others or conversely will unreasonably seek to prevent others from doing things.
- Rigid and stubborn in outlook, whilst also pedantic about doing the right thing.

Paranoid Personality Disorder

- Extremely sensitive to experiencing failure or rejection
- Hold grudges against people and will refuse to forgive insults, injuries or slights
- Very suspicious and will often misconstrue the friendly or neutral behavior of other people as being unfriendly or hostile. Also constantly suspicious about the fidelity of sexual partners
- A preoccupation with personal rights and a sense of these being infringed even when this is not so. Often self centered and self important
- Prone to believing in conspiracy theories about events affecting their own lives and in the world at large.

Schizoid Personality Disorder

- Find pleasure in few, if any, aspects of their life
- Unemotional, seem to be cold and unfeeling and find it very difficult to express anger or warmth to other people
- Unaffected by the praise or criticism of others and noticeably insensitive to the norms and conventions held by society
- Prefer to be on their own and have little interest in relationships (including close friendships or sexual ones)
- Very introspective and preoccupied with fantasy.

Schizotypal Personality Disorder

- Behavior is cold and aloof and in other respects is regarded as strange and eccentric.
- Experience difficulty in maintaining relationships and will tend to be socially withdrawn
- Hold unusual beliefs such as magical thinking which will influence the way they behave
- Hold ideas that are paranoid and overly suspicious
- Given to thinking obsessively about a subject without being able to let go, often this will be of a sexual or violent nature.

- Unusual perceptions such as 'voices', 'visions', 'bodily experiences'. Sometimes experienced as intense 'psychotic' episodes .

Treatments and Self Management Strategies

Medication (pharmacological treatments): Short-term treatments may include anxiolytic or neuroleptic drugs which are given for short periods or at times of severe stress. Long-term treatments may involve the use of neuroleptics which can be helpful in cases of paranoid and schizotypal personality disorders. However, it is possible that the medication is being used to control risk and stress, rather than having any long-term impact on the personality disorder itself.

Psychodynamic treatment: This treatment emphasizes personality structure and development. It aims to provide insight for people allowing them to understand their feelings and to find better coping mechanisms. This approach has had limited success and is likely to be less successful for those with addiction and/or antisocial personality disorder.

Cognitive and behavioral therapy: Cognitive and behavioral therapies cover a wide range of treatments such as cognitive therapy, dialectical behavior therapy, interpersonal psychotherapy and cognitive analytic therapy. Most cognitive behavioral approaches address specific aspects of thoughts, feelings, behavior or attitude, and do not claim to treat the entire personality disorder of the person. Research suggests that there are some short-term benefits to these approaches but more research is required into the long-term benefits.

Therapeutic communities: The therapeutic community (TC) approach involves living in a therapeutic community for several months. Engagement in therapy is voluntary and responsibility for the day to day running of the TC is shared between patients and staff. Members of the TC are encouraged to talk about their feelings, and particularly their feelings about each others' behavior. This encourages them to think about the affect of their own behavior on other people. The results of TC are still under scrutiny.

Chapter 10

Psychosexual Disorders

THE SEXUAL RESPONSE CYCLE

The sexual response cycle refers to the sequence of physical and emotional changes that occur as a person becomes sexually aroused and participates in sexually stimulating activities, including intercourse and masturbation. Knowing how your body responds during each phase of the cycle can enhance your relationship and help you pinpoint the cause of any sexual problems.

The Phases of the Sexual Response Cycle

The sexual response cycle has four phases: Excitement, plateau, orgasm, and resolution. Both men and women experience these phases, although the timing usually is different. For example, it is unlikely that both partners will reach orgasm at the same time. In addition, the intensity of the response and the time spent in each phase varies from person to person. Understanding these differences may help partners better understand one another's bodies and responses, and enhance the sexual experience.

Phase 1: Excitement

General characteristics of the excitement phase, which can last from a few minutes to several hours, include the following:
- Muscle tension increases.
- Heart rate quickens and breathing is accelerated.
- Skin may become flushed (blotches of redness appear on the chest and back).
- Nipples become hardened or erect.
- Blood flow to the genitals increases, resulting in swelling of the woman's clitoris and labia minora (inner lips), and erection of the man's penis.
- Vaginal lubrication begins.
- The woman's breasts become fuller and the vaginal walls begin to swell.
- The man's testicles swell, his scrotum tightens, and he begins secreting a lubricating liquid.

Phase 2: Plateau

General characteristics of the plateau phase, which extends to the brink of orgasm, include the following:
- The changes begun in phase 1 are intensified.
- The vagina continues to swell from increased blood flow, and the vaginal walls turn a dark purple.

- The woman's clitoris becomes highly sensitive (may even be painful to touch) and retracts under the clitoral hood to avoid direct stimulation from the penis.
- The man's testicles are withdrawn up into the scrotum.
- Breathing, heart rate, and blood pressure continue to increase.
- Muscle spasms may begin in the feet, face, and hands.
- Muscle tension increases.

Phase 3: Orgasm

The orgasm is the climax of the sexual response cycle. It is the shortest of the phases and generally lasts only a few seconds. General characteristics of this phase include the following:
- Involuntary muscle contractions begin.
- Blood pressure, heart rate, and breathing are at their highest rates, with a rapid intake of oxygen.
- Muscles in the feet spasm.
- There is a sudden, forceful release of sexual tension.
- In women, the muscles of the vagina contract. The uterus also undergoes rhythmic contractions.
- In men, rhythmic contractions of the muscles at the base of the penis result in the ejaculation of semen.
- A rash, or "sex flush" may appear over the entire body.

Phase 4: Resolution

During resolution, the body slowly returns to its normal level of functioning, and swelled and erect body parts return to their previous size and color. This phase is marked by a general sense of well-being, enhanced intimacy and, often, fatigue. Some women are capable of a rapid return to the orgasm phase with further sexual stimulation and may experience multiple orgasms. Men need recovery time after orgasm, called a refractory period, during which they cannot reach orgasm again. The duration of the refractory period varies among men and usually lengthens with advancing age.

Normal sexuality is difficult to define. But it is easier to define abnormal sexuality. Sexual behavior is diverse and determined by a complex interaction of factors. It is affected by relationships with others, by life circumstances, and by the culture in which a person lives. Humans, like other animals, have always been interested in sexuality and have depicted almost every form of sexual behavior.

Sexual dysfunctions are cognitive, affective, and/or behavioral problems that prevent an individual or couple from engaging in and/or enjoying satisfactory intercourse and orgasm. Sexual dysfunctions are also seen as disturbances in one more of the sexual response cycle's phases, or pain associated with arousal or intercourse. Sexual dysfunction refers to a person's inability to participate in a sexual relationship as he or she would wish.

Classification: (DSM IV TR)

Sexual desire disorder
- Hypoactive sexual desire disorder
- Sexual aversion disorder

Sexual arousal disorder
- Female sexual arousal disorder
- Male erectile disorder

Orgasmic disorder
- Female orgasmic disorder
- Male orgasmic disorder
- Premature ejaculation

Sexual pain disorder
- Vaginisumns
- Dyspareunia

Sexual dysfunction due to a general medical condition.

Types

Sexual Desire Disorders

a. **Hypoactive sexual desire disorder:** It is characterized by a persistent or recurrent deficiency or absence of sexual fantasies and desire for sexual activity. The complaint is more common in women than in men.

b. **Sexual aversion disorder:** This disorder is characterized by a persistent or recurrent extreme aversion to, and avoidance of, all genital sexual contact with a sexual partner. Individuals displaying hypoactive desire are often neutral or indifferent toward sexual interaction, but sexual aversion implies anxiety, fear or disgust in sexual situations.

Sexual Arousal Disorder

a. **Female sexual arousal disorder:** It is characterized by the persistent or recurrent partial or complete failure to attain or maintain the lubrication swelling response of sexual excitement until the completion of the sexual act.

b. **Male erectile disorder :** It is characterized by the recurrent and persistent, partial or complete failure to attain or maintain an erection to perform the sex act. Primary erectile dysfunction refers to cases in which the man has never been able to have intercourse. Secondary erectile dysfunction refers to cases in which the man has difficulty getting or maintaining an erection but has been able to have vaginal or anal intercourse at least once.

Orgasmic Disorders

a. **Female orgasmic disorder:** It is characterized by persistent or recurrent delay in, or absence of, orgasm following a normal sexual excitement phase. In short, a women's inability to achieve organism by masturbation or coitus.

Primary orgasmic dysfunction: Never experienced orgasm by any kind of stimulation.

Secondary orgasmic dysfunction: Experienced at least one orgasm, regardless of the means of stimulation, but no longer does so. Sometimes referred to as an anorgasmia.

b. ***Male orgasmic disorder :*** It is characterized by persistent or recurrent delay in, or absence of orgasm following a normal sexual excitement phase. Sometimes called retarded ejaculation A man with lifelong orgasmic disorder was never been able to ejaculate during coitus.

Primary disorder: History of never having experienced an orgasm.

Secondary disorder: Occasional problems in ejaculation.

c. ***Premature ejaculation:*** It is described as persistent or recurrent ejaculation with minimal sexual stimulation before, on, or shortly after penetration and before the person wishes it.

35–40% of men treated for sexual disorders have premature ejaculation as the chief complaints.

Sexual Pain Disorders

a. ***Dyspareunia:*** It is recurrent or persistent genital pain occurring in either men or women before, during, or after intercourse. More common in women. It is related to, and often coincides with, vaginismus. In women, the pain may be felt in the vagina, around the vaginal entrance and clitoris, or deep in the pelvis. In men, the pain is felt in the penis.

b. ***Vaginismus:*** It is an involuntary constriction of the outer one third of the vagina that prevents penile insertion and intercourse.

Sexual Dysfunction due to a General Medical Condition and Substance induced Sexual Dysfunction

Types of medical conditions that are associated with sexual dysfunction include; neurological (multiple sclerosis, neuropathy) endocrine (diabetes mellitus, thyroid dysfunctions) vascular (atherosclerosis) genitourinary (testicular disease, urethral or vaginal infections). Substances (alcohol, amphetamines, cocaine, opioids, sedatives, hypnotics, anxiolytics, antidepressants, antipsychotics and antihypertensive).

Etiology

1. ***Psychological causes:*** Stress or anxiety from work or family responsibilities, concern about sexual performance, conflicts in the relationship with partner. Depression/anxiety unresolved sexual orientation issues. Previous traumatic sexual or physical experience, body image and self esteem problems.
2. ***Physical causes:*** Diabetes, hearts disease, liver disease, kidney disease, pelvic surgery, pelvic injury or trauma, neurological disorders, medication side effects, hormonal changes, alcohol or drug abuse and fatigue.

3. *Interpersonal relationship:* Partner performance and technique, lack of partner relationship quality and conflict, lack of privacy.
4. *Sociocultural*
   - Inadequate education
   - Conflict with religious, personal or family values
   - Societal taboos.

Treatment

Basic principles of direct treatment of sexual dysfunction
- Mutual responsibility information and education attitude change
- Eliminating performance anxiety increasing communication and effectiveness of sexual technique
- Changing destructive life styles and sex roles
- Prescribing changes in behavior.

Biological Treatment

a. **Pharmacotherapy:** Sildenafil, oral phentolamine, alprostadil transurethral alprostadil (erectile disorder). Intravenous methohexital sodium has been used in desensitization therapy. Antianxiety agents, bromocriptive, a dopamine agonist, may improve sexual function impaired by hyperprolocatinemia. Dopaminergic agents have been reported to increase libido and improve sex function.
b. **Hormone therapy:** Androgens increase the sex drive. Antiandrogens have been used to treat compulsive sexual behavior in men. Antiestrogens increases libido.
c. **Mechanical treatment approaches:**

   Vacuum pump:
   These are mechanical devices that patients without vascular diseases can use to obtain erections. The blood drawn into the penis following the creation of the vacuum is kept there by a ring placed around the base of the penis.

   EROS: A device developed to create clitoral erections in women. It is a small suction cup that fits over the clitoral region and drawn blood into the clitoris.
d. **Surgical treatment:** Male prostheses vascular surgery hymenectomy for dyspareunia vaginoplasty and release of vaginal adhesions.

Dual Sex Therapy: (William Masters and Virginia Johnson)

Treatment is based on a concept that the couple must be treated when a dysfunctional person is in a relationship, both are involved in a sexually distressing situation, both must participate in the therapy program. The keystone of the program is the round table session in which a male and female therapy team clarifies, discusses, and works through problems with the couple. Treatment is short-term and behaviorally oriented. Therapist suggests specific sexual activities. Initially, intercourse is inter directed and the couple learn to give and receive

bodily pleasure without the pressure of performance or penetration. The aim of the therapy is to establish an effective communication within the marital unit. Psychotherapy sessions follow each new exercise period, and problems and satisfactions are discussed.

Specific Techniques of Exercises

Vaginismus: Woman is advised to dilate her vaginal opening with her fingers or with dilators premature ejaculation:

a. *Squeeze technique* is used to raise the threshold of penile excitability. In this exercise, the man or the woman stimulates the erect penis until the earliest sensations of impending ejaculation are felt. At this point, the woman forcefully sequeezes the coronal ridge of the gland, the erection is diminished, and ejaculation is inhibited.

b. *Stop start technique* in which the woman stops all stimulation of the penis when the man first senses an impending ejaculation.
Erectile disorder: Sometimes told to masturbate to prove that full erection and ejaculation are possible.
Lifelong female orgasmic disorder: Women is directed to masturbate, sometimes using a vibrator.

c. *Hypnotherapy*: Focus specifically on the anxiety producing situation—that is, the sexual interaction that results in dysfunction.

d. *Behavior therapy:* Behavior therapists assume that sexual dysfunction is learned maladaptive behavior, which causes patients to be fearful of sexual interaction. Hierarchy of anxiety provoking situations. Ranging from least threatening to most threatening systematic desensitization assertiveness training.

e. *Group therapy*: Used to examine both intrapsychic and interpersonal problems in patients with sexual disorders. Groups can be organized in several ways.

f. *Analytically oriented sex therapy*: The sex therapy is conducted over a longer period than usual, which allows learning or relearning of sexual satisfaction under the realities of patient's day-to-day lives.

Chapter 11
Childhood Mental Disorders

Child psychiatry is concerned with the assessment and treatment of children's emotional and behavioral problems. These problems are very common with prevalence rates of 10–20% in several community studies. Psychological disturbance in childhood is most usefully defined as an abnormality in at least one of three areas; emotions, behavior or relationships.

In childhood, the distinction between disturbance and normality is often imprecise or arbitrary. Isolated symptoms are common and not pathological. Another distinctive feature of childhood psychiatric disturbance is that several factors rather than one contribute to the development of disturbance. Etiological factors are usually categorized into two groups, constitutional and environmental. The former include hereditary factors, intelligence and temperament. The three major environmental influences are the family schooling and the community. Another factor physical illness or disability, if present can have a profound effect on the child's development and on his vulnerability to disturbance.

Three other considerations are of general importance in understanding children's behavior:
- The situationspecific nature of behavior
- The impact of current stressful life circumstances, and
- The role of the family.

Cause of Psychiatric Disturbance

Three main factors are identified:
Constitutional
- Genetic
- Temperamental
- Intrauterine disease or damage
- Birth trauma.

Environmental
- Family
- School
- Community

Physical damage or illness
- Especially neurological disease.

Classification

DSM-IV-TR and ICD-10 classification systems (modified for child psychiatry)

DSM-IV-TR	ICD-10
Axis 1 • Clinical syndrome Axis 2 • Mental retardation • Pervasive developmental disorders • Specific developmental disorders Axis 3 • Physical disorders/illness Axis 4 • Severity of current • Psychosocial stressors Axis 5 • Highest level of adaptive functioning in past year	Axis 1 • Clinical syndrome Axis 2 • Disorders of psychological development Axis 3 • Mental retardation Axis 4 • Medical illness Axis 5 • Abnormal psychosocial conditions Axis 6 • Psychosocial disability

Clinical syndromes of DSM-IV-TR and ICD-10

DSM-IV-TR	ICD-10
Axis 1 Disruptive behavior disorders • Attention deficit hyperactivity disorder (ADHD) • Conduct disorder • Oppositional defiant disorder Anxiety disorders of childhood or adolescence • Separation anxiety disorder • Avoidant disorder of childhood and adolescence • Over anxious disorder Eating disorders • Anorexia nervosa • Bulimia nervosa • Pica • Rumination disorder of infancy Gender disorders Tic disorders Elimination disorders • Functional encopresis • Functional enuresis Miscellaneous disorders **Axis 2** Pervasive developmental disorders	**Axis 1** Conduct disorders Emotional disorders Mixed disorders of conduct and emotions Hyperkinetic disorders Disorders of social functioning Tic disorders Pervasive developmental disorders Other behavioral and emotional disorders

Causative factors in childhood disturbances (epidemiological research findings)

Family discord
- Marital discord
- Children in care
- Children not living with both natural parents

Parental deviance
- Psychiatric disorder in the mother
- Criminal record in the father

Social disadvantage
- Large family size
- Overcrowding
- Father in unskilled occupation

Schooling
- High pupil/staff ratio
- High turnover of teachers.

Assessment Procedures

Assessment is more time consuming in child psychiatry than in other branches of psychiatry or medicine. It has three components:
- The diagnostic assessment interview
- Psychological assessment
- Information about the child and parents from other professionals.

MENTAL RETARDATION

Definition

Mental retardation is defined as significantly sub-average or below average general intellectual functioning, associated with deficit or impairment in adaptive functioning, which manifests during the developmental period (before 18 years of age).

General intellectual function means the result of a standardized intelligence test.

Adaptive behaviors is the person's ability to meet the responsibilities of social, personal, occupational and interpersonal areas of life according to his or her age and sociocultural and educational background.

Mental retardation is otherwise known as mental sub-normality or mental deficiency or mentally handicap.

Growth and development is slow in mentally retarded children. Mentally retarded children can have associated conditions like fits, hearing, visual or physical handicap or behavioral problems.

Incidence: 1 to 2% of the general population is mentally retard.

Causes

1. **Prenatal (Probably in 5% of cases)**
   - Infection, e.g. rubella, syphiter, toxoplasmosis, aids
   - Material disease, e.g. DM, HT, malnutrition, hypothyroidism
   - Drugs during first trimester (drugs, alcohol)
   - Physical damage, e.g. injury, radiation, hypoxia
   - Genetic.
- Inborn errors of metabolism, e.g. phenylketonuria, homocystinuria (amino acid) Tay-Sachs disease, Gaucher's disease (lipid)
- Galactosemia, glycogen storage disease (CH_2O)

- Single gene disorders, e.g. tuberous sclerosis
- Cranial anomalies, e.g. microcephly.
1. **Natal causes:** Premature birth, low birth weight, lack of respiration immediately after birth, hypoxia, birth asphyxia, birth trauma, intrauterine growth retardation, kernicterus, placental abnormalities, intraventricular hemorrhage.
2. **Postnatal cause:** Infection, e.g. encephalitis meningitis, malnutrition, cretinism, trauma (any brain injury), repeated fits.
3. **Sociocultural causes (probably in 15% of cases)**
4. **Psychiatric disorders (Probably in 1–2% of cases):** Infantile autism and childhood onset schizophrenia.

Important causes: Phenylketonuria, Down's syndrome, tuberous sclerosis, fragile X syndrome, cretinism, cerebral palsy.

Phenylketonuria

- It is the inborn error of metabolism.
- It accounts for 0.5–1% of all cases of MR
- It is an autosomal recessive disorder.

The basic defect is the absence or inactivity of phenylalanine hydronylase, a hepatic enzyme, responsible for catalysis of phenylalanine to para-tyrosine conversion. It results in marked increase in blood phenylalanine levels and it metabolites.

Clinical features: Short stature, widely spared upper incisors, epilepsy, hyperactivity, poor communication skills and poor motor coordination.

Diagnostic Evaluation

Fernic chloride test—Addition of $FeCl_3$ to urine gives a green color in patients of phenylketonuria. This results form the presence of phenylpyruvic acid in urine.
Guthrie's test—This involves a backeriological procedure aimed at measurement of phenylalanine levels in blood.

Treatment

Low phenylalanine diet best started before the age of 6 months and usually continued up to 5–6 years of age. The diet should not be completely devoid of phenylalanine, and it is an essential amino acid and its absence may itself be hazardous.

Down Syndrome (Mongolism)

It occurs in 1 out of every 700 births. It accounts for about 10% of moderate to severe mentally retarded children.
Etiology: Higher maternal age (more than 35 years).
Clinical features: Hypotonia, hyperflexibility, round face, flat nasal bridge, short ears, congenital heart disease (in about 35% of cases), gastrointestinal anomalies

(in 10%), chronic serous otitis media (in more than 50%), hypothroidism, Alzheimer disease (in 30 to 40%), epilepsy (in about 10%), loose skin folds at the nape of neck, high arched palate, thick tongue, incurved little fingers.

Tuberous Sclerosis (Epiloia)

It is autosomal dominant disorders.
Clinical features: Known as Vogt's triad
- Mental retardation, ranging from mild to severe
- Convulsions
- Adenoma sebaceum, present on face (usually red) and also on rest of the body (usually brownish white). The distribution on face is usually of butterfly type.

Fragile X Syndrome

It is the second commonest chromosomal aberration causing MR occurring in 1 out of 1000 live births.
Clinical feature: Short stature, large head, large ear, long face, big sized testes (after puberty), psychiatric disorders like attention deficit disorders.

Cretinism

Goitrous cretinism is a common cause of MR.
Clinical features: Goiter, dwarfism, coarse skin, ossification delay, apathy, hoarseness of voice, large tongue, subnormal temperature, pot belly, anemia, hypotonia of muscles.

Cerebral Palsy

Mental retardation is present in about 70% of all cases and ranges from mild to severe common feature of paralysis of limbs. Paralysis may be monoplegia, hemiplegia, paraplegia, triplegia or quadriplegia.

COMMON TYPES OF BEHAVIOR PROBLEMS WITH MENTAL RETARDATION

- Hyperactive—restlessness, running excessive talking
- Conduct disorders—disobedience, stubbornness, temper tantam poor frustration tolerance, excessive demanding
- Violent, destructive and disruptive behavior—pushing, beating, biting, damage article, shouting
- Self-injurious behavior—beating self, self-biting
- Sterotyped behavior
- Autistic behavior
- Antisocial behavior
- Dangerous behavior—fire, play with knives
- Sleep related problem
- Eating/feeding problem

- Affective disturbance—excessive crying, irritability, apathy, anger.
- Sexually inappropriate behavior
- Other odd behavior—touching others unnecessarily, standing too close to other, kissing, spiting.

CLASSIFICATION OF MENTAL RETARDATION

Mild mental retardation (IQ range 50–70)
- This is the commonest type of MR accounting for 85–90% of all cases.
- In the pre-school period (before 5 years of age), these children often develop like other normal children with very little deficit.
- Latter, the often progress upto 6th class in school and can achieve vocational and social self sufficiency with a little support.
- This group has been referred to as 'educable'.

Moderate mental retardation (IQ range 35–50)
- About 10% of all mentally retarded have an IQ between 35 to 50.
- They drop out of school after the 2nd class.
- They can be trained to support themselves by performing semi-skilled or unskilled work up under supervision.
- This group has been referred to as 'trainable'.

Profound mental retardation (IQ less than 20)
- It accounts for 1–2% of all mentally retarded.
- The achievement of development milestones is markedly delayed.
- They need nursing care or life support under a carefully planned and structured environment like group homes.

Myths and Misconceptions about Mental Retardation

Myth: Mental retardation is a hereditary problem.
Fact: Only a few causes of mental retardation are hereditary, i.e. passed on from parents to children. Mental retardation is often caused by external influences, some of which can be prevented.

Myth: Bad deeds in the previous life of parents cause mental retardation.
Fact: This is completely false. Such beliefs add to the suffering of the families who are already overburdened with caring for their special children. Some communities perpetuate the myth that if one tries to remedy the illness or take treatment, the suffering will be repeated in one's next life. This results in added suffering to the patient from lack of proper treatment.

Myth: Mental retardation is caused by pregnant and lactating women not following restrictions on food.
Fact: Pregnant and lactating women must maintain good nutrition for their own health and also for the health of the unborn or newly-born child. There is absolutely no basis for restricting food to pregnant and lactating women. However, some medications, if taken during pregnancy, may lead to malformations in the unborn child. Medication should be taken only on the prescription of a doctor. When consulting a doctor for an illness, women should always inform the doctor about being pregnant.

Contd...

Contd...

Myth: Mental retardation is caused by pregnant and lactating women not following restrictions on food.
Fact: Pregnant and lactating women must maintain good nutrition for their own health and also for the health of the unborn or newly-born child. There is absolutely no basis for restricting food to pregnant and lactating women. However, some medications, if taken during pregnancy, may lead to malformations in the unborn child. Medication should be taken only on the prescription of a doctor. When consulting a doctor for an illness, women should always inform the doctor about being pregnant.

Myth: Mental retardation is infectious.
Fact: This is completely false. Mental retardation cannot be spread by touching a patient. Children with mental retardation must be cuddled and loved just as much as normal healthy children.

Myth: Tonics/vitamins/medicines can cure mental retardation.
Fact: If mental retardation is caused by a treatable condition, appropriate treatment will cure it. However, there are no "brain tonics" which can stimulate a damaged brain. Many unscrupulous healers and manufacturers market such substances with popular and misleading names, which imply that if these substances are taken, the child will become normal. This is particularly common in rural areas, where quacks market some mixtures, guaranteeing parents a cure. These substances frequently contain a substance called 'steroids'. These medications make the child plumper and perhaps happier temporarily, which makes the parents feel good. But the basic condition of mental retardation is not cured. In fact, steroids are harmful if taken for long durations.

Myth: Brain operations can cure mental retardation.
Fact: There are very few conditions leading to mental retardation which can be cured by surgery.

Myth: Marriage can cure mental retardation.
Fact: This is completely false. In fact, a mentally retarded person should be married only with the full consent and knowledge of the partner.

Myth: Children with mental retardation become completely normal when they grow up to be adults.
Fact: Children can make substantial progress as they grow up. However, it is unlikely that they will become completely normal. Each case must be assessed individually.

Myth: Mentally retarded adults have poor sexual control and pose a danger to others.
Fact: In fact, adults with mental retardation are sexually more inhibited than their normal counterparts. On the contrary, many such people are victims of sexual abuse.

Myth: Mentally retarded children are incapable of learning anything and so everything has to be done for them.
Fact: These children are capable of learning, although how much they learn and at what speed they learn may vary. The harder we work with them, the more they will learn and more independent they can become. There is no better solution to their development than working hard with them.

Myth: Mentally retarded children should not be made to cry for any reason or should not be disciplined in any fashion.
Fact: All children need to be disciplined. Every effort should be made to teach children with mental retardation what is right and what is wrong, recognizing their capacity for learning and taking into consideration factors beyond their control.

Myth: Faith healers can cure mental retardation.
Fact: This is completely untrue. There are many sad stories about parents selling all their valuables and their land on the advice of faith healers and giving this away in charity, frequently to the faith healer. Faith healers mislead the parents. There are many alternative systems of medicine practiced in SEAR Member Countries, some of which claim to have a 'cure' for mental retardation. However, considerable research is still needed before their exact efficacy and safety can be established.

Management

Primary Prevention

  i. Improvement in socioeconomic condition of society at large aiming at elimination of under stimulation, prematurity and perinatal factors.
  ii. Education of lay public, aiming at removal of misconceptions about mentally retarded individuals.
  iii. Medical measures for good perinatal medical care to prevent infections trauma, excessive use of medication, malnutrition, obstetric complications and diseases of pregnancy.
  iv. Facilitating research activities to study the causes of mental reladation and their treatment.
  v. Genetic counseling in at-risk parents, e.g. phenylketonuria Down syndrome.

Secondary Prevention

  i. Early detection and treatment of preventable disorders, e.g. phenylketonuria (low phenylalanine diet) maple syrup urine disease (low branched amino-acid hypothyroidism (thyroxin).
  ii. Early detection of handicaps in sensor, motor or behavioral areas with early remedical measures and treatment.
  iii. Early treatment of correctable disorders, e.g. infection – antibiotics
  iv. Early recognition of presence of mental retardation. A delay in diagnosismay cause unfortunate delay in rehabilitation.

Tertiary Prevention

  i. Treatment of psychological and behavioral problems
  ii. Behavior modification
  iii. Rehabilitation in vocational, physicals and social areas
  iv. Parental counseling
  v. Institutionalization
  vi. Health education regarding MR.

As far as possible the mentally retarded children should be taken care of at home, so that they get emotional support.

- MR cannot be cured but can be improved through proper care
- MR children improve with training, but slowly.
  - Good food, love and affection
  - Special education and training
  - Good social support
- Medicines cannot cure mental retardation, but complication such as behavioral problems and epilepsy can be effectively controlled by them.
- The goal of rehabilitation of the MR is to make them an independent as possible.
- Marriage is not a cure for mental retardation. Moderate to severely retarded persons cannot take the responsibilities of marital life.

Parent's Counseling

The parents of mentally retarded children requires lifelong adjustment. Hence, the parents need guidance and counseling which is an important aspect of the management of the mentally retarded. This will help the parents to understand and to accept the child's problems and in making plans according to the capacity of the mentally retarded person.

Counseling should focus on:
a   Giving information regarding the condition of the mentally retarded child.
b. Developing the right attitude towards the handicapped child.
c. Educating the parents regarding their role in the training of the retarded child.

DIFFERENCE IN MENTAL RETARDATION AND MENTAL ILLNESS

Mental illness is a disease which can be cured. Mental retardation is developmental disorders in which there is impaired ability. So MR is not a disease. It cannot be cured. However, the associated conditions like deafness, poor vision and emotional disturbances can be treated. So, the handicap can be reduced.

AUTISM SPECTRUM DISORDERS

Autism spectrum disorders (ASDs) are a group of developmental disabilities that can cause significant social, communication and behavioral challenges. People with ASDs handle information in their brain differently than other people.

ASDs are "spectrum disorders." That means ASDs affect each person in different ways, and can range from very mild to severe. People with ASDs share some similar symptoms, such as problems with social interaction. But there are differences in when the symptoms start, how severe they are, and the exact nature of the symptoms.

Types of ASDs

There are three different types of ASDs:
- **Autistic Disorder (also called "classic" autism):** This is what most people think of when hearing the word "autism". People with autistic disorder usually have significant language delays, social and communication challenges, and unusual behaviors and interests. Many people with autistic disorder also have intellectual disability.
- **Asperger Syndrome:** People with Asperger syndrome usually have some milder symptoms of autistic disorder. They might have social challenges and unusual behaviors and interests. However, they typically do not have problems with language or intellectual disability.
- **Pervasive Developmental Disorder-Not Otherwise Specified (PDD-NOS; also called "atypical autism"):** People who meet some of the criteria for autistic disorder or Asperger syndrome, but not all, may be diagnosed with

PDD-NOS. People with PDD-NOS usually have fewer and milder symptoms than those with autistic disorder. The symptoms might cause only social and communication challenges.

Signs and Symptoms

ASDs begin before the age of 3 and last throughout a person's life, although symptoms may improve over time. Some children with an ASD show hints of future problems within the first few months of life. In others, symptoms might not show up until 24 months or later. Some children with an ASD seem to develop normally until around 18 to 24 months of age and then they stop gaining new skills, or they lose the skills they once had.

A person with an ASD might:
- Not respond to their name by 12 months
- Not point at objects to show interest (point at an airplane flying over) by 14 months
- Not play "pretend" games (pretend to "feed" a doll) by 18 months
- Avoid eye contact and want to be alone
- Have trouble understanding other people's feelings or talking about their own feelings
- Have delayed speech and language skills
- Repeat words or phrases over and over (echolalia)
- Give unrelated answers to questions
- Get upset by minor changes
- Have obsessive interests
- Flap their hands, rock their body, or spin in circles
- Have unusual reactions to the way things sound, smell, taste, look, or feel.

Treatment

There is currently no cure for ASDs. However, research shows that early intervention treatment services can greatly improve a child's development. Early intervention services help children from birth to 3 years old (36 months) learn important skills. Services can include therapy to help the child talk, walk, and interact with others. Therefore, it is important to talk to your child's doctor as soon as possible if you think your child has an ASD or other developmental problem.

Even if your child has not been diagnosed with an ASD, he or she may be eligible for early intervention treatment services. The Individuals with Disabilities Education Act (IDEA) says that children under the age of 3 years (36 months) who are at risk of having developmental delays may be eligible for services. These services are provided through an early intervention system in your state. Through this system, you can ask for an evaluation.

In addition, treatment for particular symptoms, such as speech therapy for language delays, often does not need to wait for a formal ASD diagnosis.

ATTENTION DEFICIT HYPERACTIVITY DISORDER

The Attention Deficit Hyperactivity Disorder (ADHD) is one of the most common neurobehavioral disorders of childhood. It is usually first diagnosed in childhood and often lasts into adulthood. Children with ADHD have trouble paying attention, controlling impulsive behaviors (may act without thinking about what the result will be), and in some cases, are overly active.

Signs and Symptoms

It is normal for children to have trouble focusing and behaving at one time or another. However, children with ADHD do not just grow out of these behaviors. The symptoms continue and can cause difficulty at school, at home, or with friends.

A child with ADHD might:
- Have a hard time paying attention
- Daydream a lot
- Not seem to listen
- Be easily distracted from schoolwork or play
- Forget things
- Be in constant motion or unable to stay seated
- Squirm or fidget
- Talk too much
- Not be able to play quietly
- Act and speak without thinking
- Have trouble taking turns
- Interrupt others.

Myths about attention deficit disorder	
Myth	Fact
All kids with ADD/ADHD are hyperactive.	Some children with ADD/ADHD are hyperactive, but many others with attention problems are not. Children with ADD/ADHD who are inattentive, but not overly active, may appear to be spacey and unmotivated.
Kids with ADD/ADHD can never pay attention.	Children with ADD/ADHD are often able to concentrate on activities they enjoy. But no matter how hard they try, they have trouble maintaining focus when the task at hand is boring or repetitive.
Kids with ADD/ADHD choose to be difficult and could behave better if they wanted to.	Children with ADD/ADHD may do their best to be good, but still be unable to sit still, stay quiet, or pay attention. They may appear disobedient, but that does not mean they're acting out on purpose.
Kids will eventually grow out of ADD/ADHD.	ADD/ADHD often continues into adulthood, so do not wait for your child to outgrow the problem. Treatment can help your child learn to manage and minimize the symptoms.
Medication is the best treatment option for ADD/ADHD.	Medication is often prescribed for attention deficit disorder, but it might not be the best option for your child. Effective treatment for ADD/ADHD also includes education, behavior therapy, support at home and school, exercise, and proper nutrition.

Types

There are three different types of ADHD, depending on which symptoms are strongest in the individual:
- **Predominantly Inattentive Type:** It is hard for the individual to organize or finish a task, to pay attention to details, or to follow instructions or conversations. The person is easily distracted or forgets details of daily routines.
- **Predominantly Hyperactive-Impulsive Type:** The person fidgets and talks a lot. It is hard to sit still for long (e.g. for a meal or while doing homework). Smaller children may run, jump or climb constantly. The individual feels restless and has trouble with impulsivity. Someone who is impulsive may interrupt others a lot, grab things from people, or speak at inappropriate times. It is hard for the person to wait their turn or listen to directions. A person with impulsiveness may have more accidents and injuries than others.
- **Combined Type:** Symptoms of the above two types are equally present in the person.

Causes of ADHD

- Brain injury
- Environmental exposures (e.g. lead)
- Alcohol and tobacco use during pregnancy
- Premature delivery
- Low birth weight.

Treatment

Following are treatment options for ADHD:
- Medications
- Behavioral intervention strategies
- Parent training
- ADHD and school.

Medications

Medication can help a child with ADHD in their everyday life and may be a valuable part of a child's treatment. Medication is one option that may help better control some of the behavior problems that have led to trouble in the past with family, friends and at school.
Several different types of medications may be used to treat ADHD:
- **Stimulants** are the best-known and most widely used treatments. Between 70–80% of children with ADHD respond positively to these medications.
- **Nonstimulants** were approved for treating ADHD in 2003. This medication seems to have fewer side effects than stimulants and can last up to 24 hours.

Medications can affect children differently, where one child may respond well to one medication, but not another. When determining the best treatment, the

doctor might try different medications and doses, so it is important to work with your child's doctor to find the medication that works best for your child.

Behavioral Therapy

Research shows that behavioral therapy is an important part of treatment for children with ADHD. ADHD affects not only a child's ability to pay attention or sit still at school, it also affects relationships with family and how well they do in their classes. Behavioral therapy is another treatment option that can help reduce these problems for children and should be started as soon as a diagnosis is made. Following are examples that might help with your child's behavioral therapy:

- **Create a routine**: Try to follow the same schedule every day, from wake-up time to bedtime.
- **Get organized**: Put schoolbags, clothing, and toys in the same place every day so your child will be less likely to lose them.
- **Avoid distractions:** Turn off the TV, radio, and computer, especially when your child is doing homework.
- **Limit choices:** Offer a choice between two things (this outfit, meal, toy, etc., or that one), so that your child is not overwhelmed and overstimulated.
- **Change your interactions with your child:** Instead of long-winded explanations and cajoling, use clear, brief directions to remind your child of responsibilities.
- **Use goals and rewards:** Use a chart to list goals and track positive behaviors, then reward your child's efforts. Be sure the goals are realistic—baby steps are important!
- **Discipline effectively:** Instead of yelling or spanking, use timeouts or removal of privileges as consequences for inappropriate behavior.
- **Help your child discover a talent.** All kids need to experience success to feel good about themselves. Finding out what your child does well — whether it is sports, art, or music — can boost social skills and self-esteem.

Parent Training

Another important part of treatment for a child with ADHD is parent training. Children with ADHD may not respond to the usual parenting practices, so experts recommend parent education. This approach has been successful in educating parents on how to teach their kids about organization, develop problem-solving skills and cope with their ADHD symptoms.

Parent training can be conducted in groups or with individual families and are offered by therapists or in special classes. Children and adults with attention deficit/hyperactivity disorder (CHADD) offers a unique educational program to help parents and individuals navigate the challenges of ADHD across the lifespan.

ADHD and the Classroom

Just like with parent training, it is important for teachers to have the needed skills to help children manage their ADHD. However, since the majority of children

with ADHD are not enrolled in special education classes, their teachers will most likely be regular education teachers who might know very little about ADHD and could benefit from assistance and guidance.

Here are some tips to share with teachers for classroom success:
- Use a homework folder for parent-teacher communications
- Make assignments clear
- Give positive reinforcement
- Be sensitive to self-esteem issues
- Involve the school counselor or psychologist.

HABIT DISORDERS

Habit disorders includes tension discharging phenomena, such as—head banging, body rocking—occurring when a child is put to bed or is alone, this movements seems to provide a kind of sensory solace for the child whose is feeling otherwise uncared for or unstimulated by human touch or interaction. This movements represents a kind of internal stroking such patterns are often seen in the mentally retarded or in children suffering from maternal or emotional deprivation.

Nail biting, hair pulling (trichotillomania), thumb sucking—normal in early infancy, like other rhythmic patterns it can be seen as a way of securing extra self- nurturance.

Teeth grinding (bruxism)—seems to result from tension originating in unexpressed anger or resentment, it may create problems in dental occlusion. Helping the child to find ways to express resentment may relive the problem. Bed time can be made more enjoyable and relaxed by reading or talking with the child, permitting experience and review of some of the fears or angers experienced during the day. Praise and emotional support are useful at these times. Hitting or biting parts of once own body, body manipulations, repetitive vocalization, breath holding, swolling air (aerophagia).

Stuttering Dysfluent Speech

Primary stuttering usually begins as a atypical development during the learning of speech it starts gradually initially with the repetition of consonants, often followed by a repetition of words and phrases. Most cases resolves spontaneously and seems to remit more readily in girls. All children at various developmental points show repetitive patterns of movement that can discussed as habits. Weather they are considered as disorders depends on the degree to which interfere with child's physical, emotional, or social functioning. Some hobbit patterns may be learned by imitation of adults. Many being as a purposeful movements that, for some reason becomes repetitive, with the habit losing its original significance and becoming a means of discharging tension.

TIC DISORDER

Tic disorder are characterized by the presence of tics. Tic is an abnormal involuntary movement (AIM) which occurs repetitively, rapidly and is purposeless in nature. Symptoms begins the age of 18 years and not caused by medical condition.

Types

- Motor tic—characterized by repetitive motor movements
- Vocal tic—characterized by repetitive vocalization
- Tourette's syndrome—combined motor and vocal tics and coprolalia.

Motor Tics

Motor tics are earliest to appear, and begin in the head region progressing down wards. It can be simple or complex.
Simple motor tics: Include eye blinking, grimacing, shrugging of shoulders, tongue protrusion, head jerking.
Complex motor tics: Include stamping jumping, hitting self, squatting echo kinesis (repetition of observe acts), copropraxia (obscene acts).

Vocal Tics

Vocal tics can also be simple or complex.
Simple vocal tics: Include coughing, barking, throat clearing, sniffing, clicking.
Complex vocal tics: Include echolalia (repetition of heard pharses), palilalia (repetition of heard words), coprolalia (use of obscene words) and mental coprolalia (thinking of obscene words).

Prevalence

A large community based study suggested that over 19% of school age children have tic disorders. The children with tic disorder in that study were usually undiagnosed. As many as 1 in 100 people may experience some form of tic disorder usually before the onset of puberty.

Causes

No definitive cause of tics has been discovered.

Biological Factors

The exact neurochemical cause is unknown, it is believed that abnormal neurotransmitters like dopamine, serotonin and cyclic AMP contribute to the disorder.

Genetic Factors

Vulnerability to tic disorders appears to be genetic or transmitted within families. Genetic factors are present in 75% of cases, although no single gene has been found to cause tic disorders.

Chemical Factors

In some cases, tic disorders appear to be caused or worsened by recreational drugs or prescription medications. Drugs such as methylphenidate, pemoline, amphetamines, cocaine, etc.

Environmental Disorder

Some forms of tic may be triggered by the environment. A cough that began during an upper respiratory infection may continue as an involuntary vocal tic. New tics may also begin as imitations of normally occurring events such as mimicking a dog barking.

Treatment

A holistic approach is recommended for the treatment of tic disorder. A multidisciplinary team should work together with the affected child's parents and teachers to put together a comprehensive treatment plan.

Treatment should include the following:
- Educating the patient and family about the course of the disorder in a reassuring manner.
- Comprehensive assessment including the child's a cognitive abilities, perception, motor skills, behavior and adaptive functionary.
- Collaboration with school personnel to create a learning environment conductive to academic success.
- If necessary, evaluation for medication.

Behavioral and cognitive behavioral therapy:
- Positive reinforcement : Children are praised and rewarded for not performing tics and for replacing them with alternative behaviors.
- Self-monitoring : It is fairly effective in reducing some tics by increasing the child's awareness.
- Habit reversal is the most commonly used technique, combining relaxation exercise, awareness training and contingency management for positive reinforcement. This method shows a 64–100% success rate.

Medications:
- Antipsychotic drugs, e.g. haloperidol risperidone
- Alpha—adrenergic receptor agonists, e.g. clonidine
- SSRI, e.g. sertratine
- Benzodiazepines.

Prevention

There are few preventive strategies for tic disorders:
- There is some evidence that material emotional stress during pregnancy and severe nausea and vomiting during the first trimester may affect tic severity.
- Attempting to minimize prenatal stress may possibly serve a limited preventive function
- Attempting to maintain a low stress environment can help minimize the number or severity of tics.

CONDUCT DISORDER

Conduct disorder consists of repetitive and persistent pattern of behaviors in which the basic rights of others or major age appropriate norms or rules of society are violated.

After the age of 18, a conduct disorder may develop into anti-personality disorder. Conduct disorder is known as a disruptive behavior disorder because of its impact on children and their families, neighbors and schools.

Oppositional defiant disorder may be a precursor of conduct disorder. A child is diagnosed with oppositional defiant disorder when he or she shows signs of being hostile and defiant for at least 6 months. Oppositional defiant disorder may start as early as the preschool years, while conduct disorder generally appears when children are older.

Incidence

Conduct disorder affects 1 to 4% of 9–17 years olds. The disorder appears to be more common in boys than in girls and more common in rural areas.

Risk Factors of Conduct Disorder

- Early maternal rejection
- Separation from parents
- Early institutionalization
- Family neglect
- Abuse or violence
- Parental mental illness
- Parental marital discord
- Large family size
- Poverty.

Clinical Features

- Aggressive behavior that harms or threatens other people or animals
- Destructive behavior that damage or destroys properly
- Lying or theft
- Truancy or other serious violations of rules
- Early tobacco, alcohol and substance use and abuse
- Precocious sexual activity.

Children with conduct disorder also may experience:
- Higher rates of depression, suicidal thoughts, suicide attempts and suicide
- Academic difficulties
- Poor relationships with peers or adults
- Sexually transmitted disease
- Difficulty staying
- Higher rates of injuries, school expulsions and problems with the law.

Management

Drug treatment may be needed in presence of epilepsy (anticonvulsants), hyperactivity (stimulant medication), impulse control disorder and episodic aggressive behavior (lithium, carbamazepine) and psychotic symptoms (antipsychotic).

Child Training

- Teach new skills to facilitate the child's growth, development and adaptive functioning.
- Teach problem solving and self-control.
- Teach prosocial skills through the teaching of appropriate play skills, development of friendship and conversational skills.
- Develop cognitive skills.

School-based Programs

Teaching the child problem solving skills, strategies for increasing physiological awareness, anger management, how to be friendly, how to talk to friends and how to succeed in school.

Family Intervention

To assist parents to learn administration of appropriate reinforcement, disciplinary techniques, effective communication with the child and problem solving and negotiation strategies.

ELIMINATION DISORDER

Enuresis

Enuresis is defined as the involuntary or intentional voiding of urine either during the day or night, at inappropriate places. This condition is common in infancy. Children achieve bladder control by the age of 3 Years and still 7% children after 5 years wet their bed.

Types

- Primary enuresis—occurs when a child has never established bladder control.
- Secondary enuresis—occurs when a person has established bladder control for a period of six months, then relapses and begins wetting
- Nocturnal—passage of urine during nighttime sleep
- Diurnal—daytime wetting.

Incidence

Day time wetting is more common in girls than in boys, but bed wetting is thrice as prevalent in boys.

Causes

The exact cause of enuresis is not known
- Hormonal problems: A hormone called anti-diuretic hormone cause the body to produce less urine at night. But some people's bodies do not make enough ADH, which means their bodies may produce too much urine while they are sleeping.
- Bladder problems: In some people with enuresis, too many muscle spasms can prevent the bladder from holding a normal amount of urine. Some teens and adults also have relatively small bladders that can not hold a large volume of urine.
- Genetics: Teens with enuresis often have a parent who had the same problem at about the same age.
- Sleep problem: Some teens may sleep so deeply that they don't wake up when they need to pee.
- Medical conditions: Medical conditions that can trigger secondary enuresis include diabetes, constipation and urinary tract infections. Spiral cord trauma, sports injury, auto accident may also play a role in enuresis.
- Psychological problems such as divorce, the death of a friend or family member, insecurity, sibling rivalry.

Symptoms

The main symptoms of enuresis include
- Repeated bed wetting
- Wetting in the clothes
- Wetting at least twice a week for approximately 3 months.

Treatment

- Restriction of fluid intake after 8 PM in nocturnal enuresis
- Bladder training during daytime, aimed at increasing holding time of the bladder.
- Interruption of sleep before the expected time of bed wetting
- Conditioning devices which cause alarm to sound as soon as the voided urine touches the bed sheet. It cause inhibition of further micturation and the child awakens.
- Supportive psychotherapy to child and parents
- Pharmacotherapy with imipramine 25–75 mg/day drug of choice.

ENCOPRESIS

Encopresis is an elimination disorder that involves repeatedly having bowel movement in inappropriate places after the age when bowel control is normally expected.

Encopresis is also called 'soiling' or 'fecal in continence'.

Incidence

Encopresis is more common (3–4 times) in males. By the age of 5 years, 1–1.5% of children are encopretic. It tends to remit spontaneously with increasing age and by the age of 16, there are virtually no encopretics. 25% of these patients have associated enuresis.

Types

Primary type: Where toilet training has never been achieved.
Secondary type: Where encopresis emerges after a period of fecal continance.

Causes

- Inadequate toilet training
- Sibling rivalry
- Maturational lag
- Underlying hyperkinetic disorder
- Emotional disturbances
- Mental retardation
- Childhood schizophrenia
- Autistic disorder
- Psychological factors → shame, guilt or low self-esteem
- Damage to the internal organs, therefore unable to feel or hold feces. This is medical encopresis. It affects all the age groups.

The following may increase the risk for encopresis
- Being male
- Chronic constipation
- Low socioeconomic status.

Symptoms

- Inability to retain feces
- Passing stool in inappropriate places (generally in the child's clothes)
- Constipation and hard stools
- Occasional passage of very large stool that almost blocks up the toilet.

Treatment

- The first step to treating encopresis is to identify the cause behind the condition. It cannot be treated by scolding a child or punishing. This will only worsen the situation. Instead, a parent must reassure the child, so that he feels emotionally secure. This will encourage the child to let go of his fears and help him to master control over his bowels.
- In case of medical encopresis, it can be treated by laxative, stool softener and set time routine.
- Behavior therapy by using reinforcement.

- Psychotherapy → Enlist cooperation, show concern and develop trust
- Biofeedback
- Parent counseling/family therapy
  - Modify attitude
  - Hostile interaction
  - Secondary problems.

Treatment in Child and Adolescent Psychiatry

Drug Treatment

Drug	Usage	Comment
Anxiolytics	Anxiety/phobic conditions	Short-term adjunct to behavior treatment
Neuroleptics	Schizophrenia/hyperkinetic syndrome	
Phenothiazines, e.g. chlorpromazine Butyrophenones, e.g. Haloperidol	Complex Tics/Tourette's syndrome	Extrapyramidal side effects common
Tricyclic antidepressants		
Imipramine/amitriptyline Clomipramine	Enuresis Major affective disorder	Effective, but high relapse rate Most useful with persistent and sustained mood disturbance
Methylphenidate (Stimulants)	Hyperkinetic syndrome	Effective in the short-term. Long-term effects on growth, sleep and appetite
Fenfluramine	Pervasive developmental disorder	Effectiveness not established. Side effects include irritability, anorexia and weight loss
Hypnotics, e.g. trimeprazine/ promethazine	Persistent. Sleep disorder in preschool children	Only short-term
Lithium	Recurrent bipolar affective disorder	Close supervision of blood levels for signs of toxicity
Laxatives, e.g. bulk-forming (methylcellulose) Stimulants (senna) softener (dioctyl)	Encopresis with constipation	Facilities formation and passage of feces
Central alpha agonist, e.g. clonidine	Unresponsive Tourette's syndrome	Sedation and rebound hypertension

Behavioral Psychotherapy

Behavioral techniques
- Exposure techniques
- Desensitization
- Flooding

- Modelling
- Response prevention.

Operant Techniques
- Reinforcement
  - Positive
  - Negative
- Extinction
- Punishment
  - Application of aversive stimuli
  - Removal of reinforce
- Shaping, prompting and fading

Applications of behavior techniques

Disorder	Technique
Anxiety and phobic	Desensitization, flooding, relaxation
Obsessive-compulsive	Relaxation Relapse-prevention
Depressive disorder	Cognitive behavioural Relaxation
Conduct disorders	Positive reinforcement Extinction
Hyperactivity syndromes	Time out Positive reinforcement Extinction
Pervasive developmental disorders	Time-out Positive reinforcement Extinction Time out Aversive techniques
Encopresis/enuresis	Positive reinforcement
Mental retardation	Positive reinforcement Extinction and time-out Prompting and shaping Aversive techniques
Tics	Massed practice.

Chapter 12

Emergency Psychiatry

EMERGENCY

Emergency is defined as an unforeseen combination of circumstances which calls for immediate action.

Medical Emergency

It is defined as a condition which endangers life and/or causes great suffering to the individual patient.

Psychiatric Emergency

It is defined as a disturbance in thought, mood and/of action which causes sudden distress to the individual or other, and/or sudden disability, thus requiring immediate management.

Types of Psychiatric Emergency
- Suicide
- Stupor
- Excitement (violent)
- Refusal of food
- Delirium
- Panic attack
- Alcohol or drug dependence
  - Withdrawl syndrome
  - Overdose
  - Complication
- Deliberate harm to self or other.

SUICIDE

- Suicidology is progression from thought of suicide to attempt suicide.
- Suicide is the intentional act of killing oneself.

Suicide ideation: It means thinking about killing oneself.

Active suicidal ideation (complete suicide): When a person thinks about and seeks ways to commit suicide. It ends with fatal outcome.

Passive suicidal ideation (attempted suicide): When a person thinks about wanting to die but has no plans to commit suicide. It ends with non-fatal outcome.

Epidemiology

It is estimated that over 1,00,000 people die by suicide in India every year. India alone contributes to more than 10% of suicides in the world. Majority of suicides occur men in younger age groups. Attempted suicide is more common is women while completed suicide is common (2–4 times) in men.

Etiology

- Clients with psychiatric disorder, e.g. depression schizophrenia, substance abuse, post-traumata stress disorder, borderline personality disorder.
- Chronic medical illness, e.g. cancer, HIV/aids, head and spinal cord injury.
- Environmental factors: Isolation, any recent loss, lack of social support, unemployment, critical life events like death or a loved one, divorce, etc.
- Behavioral factors: Impulsivity and unexplained changes from usual behavior.
- Unstable lifestyle.

Risk Factors

The risk of completed suicide increases in **sad persons**. It means:

S—Sex—male
A—Age—adolescent and age more than 40 years
D—Depression—risk about 25 times more in depression than normal.
P—Previous history of suicidal attempts.
E—Ethanol—history of alcohol or drug dependence
R—Rational thinking loss due to mental illness
S—Severe illness—Presence of severe disabling, painful or untreatable physical illness
O—Organized plan—suicidal preoccupation particularly, if a 'suicide note' is written or detailed plans are made for committing suicide
N—No spouse—being unmarried, divorced, widowed or separated
S—Social isolation.

Methods Used

In India, the commonest mode of committing suicide is by ingestion of poisons (about 30%) followed by hanging (about 18%), drowning (about 18%), jumping in front of train (7%) and burning (6%).

Men use more violent methods for suicide as compared with women.

Helpful/Harmful attitudes towards a Suicidal Person
A suicidal individual feels relieved by:
  i. Someone who will listen to them—someone who has the time, who will provide undivided attention in a non-critical manner without trying to advice or intrude.
  ii. Someone whom they can trust—someone who will treat them with dignity and keep their confidentiality.

iii. Someone who shows care—someone whom they can approach, who will offer empathetic and unconditional friendship.

A suicidal individual is disturbed by:
  i. Rejection by fellow beings: Having someone to turn to make all the difference
  ii. Advices: No one like to be lectured about his/her own life
  iii. Criticism: Harsh judgment attitudes can be very hurting
  iv. Interrogative approaches: Undue probing into affairs, seeking explanation for past action etc. can further increase their mental stress.

Management of Suicidal Person

- Be direct: Talk openly and matter of factly about suicide
- Be willing to listen: Allow expression of feeling. Accept feelings
- Be non-judgmental: Do not debate if suicide is right or wrong; feelings are good or bad. Do not lecture over value of life
- Become available: Show interest and support
- Do not act shocked: This will put distance between you and the person in crisis
- Encourage to get help from persons or agencies that offer crisis support.

STUPOR

Stupor is a common condition which presents at the emergency services. The word stupor derives from the Latin word stupure meaning insensible.

Stupor is a condition where the patient is conscious, but there is non-responsiveness to the surrounding.

Etiology

- Schizophrenia (especially catatonic)
- Depression.

Clinical Feature

- Total absence of self cone
- Neglecting physiological needs like food and fluid intake
- Total motor inactivity.

Management

- Assess the nutritional states and hydration because there is risk of neglect of nutrition.
- Give immediate IV fluid
- Ryes tube-feeding can provided
- Administer vitamins to facilitate movements and to prevent contractures
- Minimal dose of drugs (antipsychotics or anti depressants) are helpful to relieve basic problems.

EXCITEMENT (VIOLENCE)

Violence is physical aggression inflicted by one person on another. They may harm others or harm themselves.

Etiology

- Psychotic disorder: Schizophrenia, mania, paranoid and postpartum psychosis
- Organic mental disorder: Delirium, drug intoxication and withdrawl
- Personality disorder: Antisocial and paranoid personality disorder
- Brain disorder: Seizure disorder, brain injury, encephalitis and MR with behavior problem.

Management

- Protect yourself, do not approach alone, call for assistance to manage any situation
- Reassure the patient
- Restraint
- This should be used as a last resort, but when needed it must not be delayed and must not be attempted in half hearted way. Restraint is usually followed by compulsory hospitalization and parenteral medication. It is rarely necessary to continue restraint for more than a few hours.
- Assess the nutritional state and if there dehydration, IV fluids are essential.
- Sedation
  The most effective drugs are:
  – Injection Chlorpromazine 100 mg
  – Injection Haloperidol 10–20 mg
  – Injection Diazepam 10 mg.

REFUSAL OF FOOD

Refusal of food may be due to the following reasons:
- They are not bothered about their nutrition (schizophrenia)
- Suspect that their food is poisoned (paranoid disorders)
- Loss of appetite, lack of interest (depression)
- Too busy and active that they do not have time to eat (mania)
- Protest against hospitalization or treatment.

Management

- Regular diet supervision
- Maintain weight chart
- Encourage and support to eat
- IV fluid or Ryle's tube-feeding if necessary.

RAPE

Rape and sexual assault are concerns for individuals, families and the community. Sexual assaults against women and children result in physical trauma, psychic and spiritual disruptions and the deterioration of social relationship.

Sexual assault is defined as forced perpetration of an act of sexual contact with another person without consent.

Silent rape reaction may be characterized as:
Loss of appetite, disturbance in sleep, fear and anxiety, social isolation, agoraphobia, fear of violence and death, pregnancy or STD.

Management

- Give reassurance to the victim
- Encourage ventilation of feeling and emotions associated with rape trauma
- Use social support system to the help the victim
- Provide reinforcement of healthy traits
- Provide adequate encouragement to return to previous level of functioning as rapidly as possible
- Do thorough physical examination
- Provide legal counseling to the victim and family
- Assess for pregnant status and provide all the alternatives to pregnancy
- Examine for veneral diseases and if found positive then administer antibiotic drugs as per order.

OTHER PSYCHOTIC EMERGENCIES

- Severe depression
- Hyperventilation syndrome
- Side effects of psychotropic medication, e.g. dystonia, akathisia, neuroleptic malignant syndromes.
  - Insomnia
  - Pseudoseizures
  - Anorexia nervosa (usually presenting with dehydration and/or cachexia)
  - Grief and bereavement
  - Psychosocial crises, e.g. marital conflict occupational and financial difficulties.

An ideal place for treating psychiatric emergencies is a separate psychiatric intensive care unit (PICU) or crisis intervention center (CIC) attached to a psychiatric unit in a general hospital or to a psychiatric hospital or nursing home.

Chapter 13
Legal Aspects of Psychiatry

The branch of the psychiatry dealing with legal aspects is forensic psychiatry. Law reflects social norms. Law comes in contact with psychiatry at many points. For example, admission of mentally ill person in a mental hospital, crime committed by a mentally ill person, validity of marriage, will, consent, right to vote, drug dependence, etc.

INDIAN LUNACY ACT (16TH MARCH 1912)

Indian Lunacy Act is derived from English Lunacy Act 1890. The Act extends to the whole of India. (expect the state of Jammu and Kashmir).
It contains eight chapters:
Chapter 1. Preliminary information
Chapter 2. Procedure for admission into a mental hospital
Chapter 3. Care, treatment and discharge
Chapter 4. Proceeding in lunacy in presidency town
Chapter 5. Proceeding in lunacy outside presidency town
Chapter 6. Establishment of asylums
Chapter 7. Expenses of lunatics
Chapter 8. Rules.

THE MENTAL HEALTH ACT-1987

The Mental Health Act 1987 replaced the Indian Lunacy Act 1912. This Act applies to whole of India including the state of Jammu and Kashmir. The Act was brought into force on 1st of April 1993.
It has 10 chapters comprising in all 98 sections:
Chapter 1. Preliminary information
Chapter 2. Mental health authorities
Chapter 3. Psychiatric hospitals and psychiatric nursing home
Chapter 4. Admission and detention in psychiatric nursing home
Chapter 5. Inspection, discharge, leave of absence and removal of mentally ill persons
Chapter 6. Judicial inquisition
Chapter 7. Liability to meet lost of maintenance of mentally ill persons
Chapter 8. Protection of human rights of mentally ill person
Chapter 9. Penalties and procedures
Chapter 10. Miscellaneous

Chapter–1: Preliminary Information

Mentally ill person: A person who is in need of treatment by reason of any mental disorder other than mental retardation (the term lunatic deleted).

Mentally ill prisoner: Means a mentally ill person for whose detention in a psychiatric hospital.

It gives information of the terms like minor, psychiatric hospital, psychiatrist, reception order, relative, etc.

Chapter–2: Mental Health Authority

It deals with the establishment of central and state mental health authority with a specified nature of work relating to regulation, development and coordination of mental health services.

Chapter–3: Psychiatric hospital and psychiatric nursing home

This chapter deals with the establishment of psychiatric hospitals and psychiatric nursing homes for the admission, treatment and care of mentally ill persons at such places as it thinks fit and separate psychiatric hospitals and psychiatric nursing homes, may be established or maintained for those who:

- Are under the age of 18 years
- Are addicted to alcohol or drug addicts
- Have been convicted of any offence
- Belong to such class or category of person as may prescribed.

Chapter–4: Admission and detention in psychiatric nursing home

Admission on voluntary basis:

- Admission would be done on voluntary approach of the patient who suffers or considers himself to suffer from a mental illness
- Any person but not a minor could seek for the said admission
- In respect of a minor, the guardian of the minor could seek for such an admission
- Whenever, such as admission in sought for the medical officer in charge of the psychiatric home or the psychiatric nursing home shall make an injury, with in the period of 24 hours and is satisfied may admit the applicant or the minor as the case may be as a voluntary inpatient.

Admission under special circumstance:

- The admission under special circumstances would arise when a mentally ill person does not or unable to express his willingness seek to admission as an impatient.
- In such of the circumstance, a relative or friend or the mentally ill person could make an application in prescribed form to the medical officer or in-charge of the psychiatric home or psychiatric nursing home.

Admission under authority or orders

- Reception orders on application:
  The Medical officer of psychiatric home, where the mentally ill person is undergoing treatment finds, that the said mentally ill person is suffering from

mental illness and requires a treatment for more than six months, or where it is found that such a detention is needed for the safety of the mentally ill person or for the protection of others such a mentally ill person should be detained, then he can make such an application for detention, before the jurisdictional magistrate where the psychiatric home is situated.

- Reception order or production of mentally ill person before magistrate:
Every officer in-charge of the police station for the reason to believe that any person within the limits of the said police station found wandering to be a mentally ill person not taking care of himself or dangerous, may take or cause to be taken that person in to protection.

So, the person who has taken in to protection and detained, shall be produced before the nearest magistrate within 24 hours of taking him into such protection.

Admission as inpatient after inquisition
The district court during an inquisition proceeding can direct that a mentally ill person shall be admitted and kept as an impatient until such time the said direction is modified or cancelled.

Admission and detention of mentally ill prisoner
- An order passed under the code of criminal procedure. Navy Act, Army Act, Air Force Act and Prisoner Act.
- The commissioner of police in the areas where is appointed could exercise the power instead of magistrate.

Chapter-5: Inspection, discharge, leave of absence and removal of mentally ill persons
Inspection: Board of visitors should visit the hospital at least once a month and atleast 3 members of the team should be present. The Director general of health services should visit once in 6 months. Whenever, the board of visitors visit the hospital, they should write remarks in the visitors book about the working of the hospital.

Discharge:
- Voluntary discharge
- Discharge under special circumstance
- Discharge in respect of admissions due to an order of an authority.

Leave of absence: The application for leave of absence should be accompanied by a bond, with or without sureties for such amount as to take proper care of the mentally ill person, to prevent the mentally ill person from causing injury to himself or to others and to bring back the mentally ill person to the psychiatric hospital.

Removal: This chapter deals with safeguarding and removal of mentally ill persons from one psychiatric hospital to another.

Chapter–6: Judicial inquisition
This deals with judicial inquisition regarding alleged mentally ill person possessing properly, custody of his person and management of his property.

Chapter–7: Liability to meet cost of maintenance of mentally ill persons

The relatives of the patients are liable to pay or to take charge of cost maintenance of the client. If they are not taking charge they are liable to pay the penalty. If the client does not have any relative or family the hospital/government will take charge of the patient.

Chapter–8: Protection of human rights of mentally ill person

It is aimed at the protection of human rights of mentally ill persons.

During the stay at hospital/when he is mentally ill, he should not be subjected to any treatment without his consent or to any indignity. No patient should be subjected to research purposes without his consent. Nothing should disturb him during his stay at hospital. Patient has right to have letter, or communication on both the sides without destroying.

Chapter–9: Penalties and procedures

If the psychiatric hospital/nursing home is not fulfilling the requirements they are liable to pay penalty. If the patient is not treated property during his stay at hospital they are liable to pay the penalty.

Chapter–10: Miscellaneous

The chapter deals with the miscellaneous rule about the conduct of the medical officer in-charge, regarding the patient and his care during his stay at hospital.

RIGHTS OF MENTALLY ILL CLIENTS

The legal and ethical context of care is important for all psychiatric nurses because it focuses concern on the rights of patients and the quality of care they receive. Psychiatric patients currently have the following rights:

- Right to communicable with people outside the hospital through correspondence, telephone and personal visits
- Right to keep clothing and personal effects with them in the hospital
- Right to religions freedom
- Right to manage and dispose of property
- Right to execute wills
- Right to privacy
- Right to informed consent
- Right to treatment
- Right to refuse treatment
- Right to civil service status.

LEGAL RESPONSIBILITIES OF A MENTALLY ILL PERSON

Criminal Responsibility

M'naghten rule: Section 84 of the Indian Penal Code of 1860 provides that "nothing is an offence which is done by a person who, at the time of doing it by reason of unsoundness of mind, was incapable of knowing the nature of the act or that what he was doing either wrong or contrary to law".

Civil Responsibility

Marriage: Under the Hindu Marriage Act (1955) a marriage between two parties, either of whom was of unsound mind at the time of the marriage is considered void. Divorce can be obtained on the ground of incurable unsoundness of mind for a specific continuous period.

The competence to be a witness: (Indian Evidence Act 1872)
An insane person is not competent to give evidence if he is prevented by his lunacy from understanding the necessity of telling the truth.

Election or right to vote: No person of unsound mind can contest an election or can vote. If he does so, it will be invalid.

Management of property and affairs of insane: On the application of any relative of an alleged lunatic, the court may direct an inquisition whether the person is of unsound mind and incapable of managing his property and affairs.

Contract: A contract is invalid if one of the parties at the time of making it was by reason of insanity was to wholly incapable of understanding what he was doing.

Consent: An unsound person who can not understand the consequences of the act can not give consent.

Testamentary Capacity: (Indian succession Act 1325), if a person suffers from mental illness at the time of making his will and if he does not have the mental capacity to understand the consequences of the act, his will becomes invalid.

THE NARCOTIC DRUGS AND PSYCHOTROPIC SUBSTANCES ACT (NDPSA) 1985

1857—The Opium Act
1878—Revised Opium Act
1930—Dangerous Drugs Act
1950—The Opium and Revenue Laws Act
1985—NDPSA

The act includes Narcotic drugs (opium, poppy, straw, cannabis, cocaine, coca and all related synthesized 'drugs') and psychotropic substances (76 drugs and their derivatives, e.g. major tranquilizers, minor tranquillizers, barbiturates, etc.). In this Act if a person produces, possesses, transports, imports, sells, purchases or uses any narcotic drugs or psychotropic substances (except Ganga) he shall be punishable with:

- Rigorous imprisonment for not less than 10 years (which may be extended upto 20 years) and a fine of not less than 1 lakh rupees (which may be extended upto 2 lakh rupees).
- For repeat offence a rigorous imprisonment for not less than 15 years (may be extended to 30 years) and a fine of not less than 1.5 lakh rupees (which may be extended upto 3 lakh rupees).

Chapter 14

Biopsychosocial Therapies

HISTORICAL DEVELOPMENT OF PSYCHOPHARMOCOLOGY

- In BC 4000, the roots of plant "serpentina mixed with oil was used in India to treat mentally ill.
- In 1853, bromide was used in treatment of mania and melancholia.
- 1882 paraldehyde used as a hypnotic.
- 1883 phenothiazines synthesized during synthesis of methiline blue.
- 1903 barbiturates (barbital) used for sedation in and phenobarbital was introduced in 1912.
- 1917 (Julius von Wagner Jauregg) used malarial treatment for General Paresis of Insane (GPI) and received Nobel Prize.
- 1922 (Jacob Klaesi) introduced barbiturate induced comma for treatment of psychosis.
- 1927 Manfred Sakel introduced insulin shock therapy in for schizophrenia
- 1931 (Ganesh Sen and Karthik Bose) reported successful treatment of psychosis using Rauwolfia Serpentina extract (reserpine).
- 1934 Laszio and Meduna in troduced metrozol-induced convulsions for treatment of psychosis.
- 1936 Egaz Moniz and Almenda Lima advocated frontal lobotomy for treatment of psychiatric disorders.
- 1937 C Bradley used amphetamine in behavioral disorders in children.
- In 1938 Ugo Cerletti and Lucio Bini introduced electroconvulsive therapy in the management of psychosis.
- 1940 Tracy Putnum used phenetoin as anticonvulant.
- 1943 Albert Hofman synthesised LSD.
- 1949 John F. Cade used lithium in mania.
- 1950 Charpentier synthesized chlorpromazine while making better anti-histaminic than promethazine.
- 1950 methyle phenindate used in the treatment of ADHD.
- 1951 Laborit used lytic cocktail in artificial hibernation.
- 1951 Isoniazid (INH) and isopiazid foud to have mood elevating properties.
- 1952 Jean Delay and Pierre Deniker) introduced chlorpromazine in the treatment of psychosis.
- 1955 meprobamate was introduced as ant-anxiety agent.
- 1958 Thomas Kuhn introduce imipramine in the treatment of depression.
- 1958 Nathan line introduced MAOIs in the management of depression.
- 1958 (Janssen) haloperidol synthesized in Belgium.

- 1960 Sternbach used chlordiazeproxide as anti-anxiety agent.
- 1966 Lambert used valproate in the treatment of bipolar disorders.
- 1968 Janssen used pimozide in the treatment of schizophrenia.
- 1967 Fernandez and Lopez-Ibor used chlomipramine in OCD.
- 1971 Takezaki and Hanoaka used carbamazepine in bipolar disorders.
- 1988 Kane et al re-discovered as an effective antipsychotic agent for refractory schizophrenia (clozapine).

ANTIPSYCHOTIC DRUGS

Antipsychotic medications are generally divided into two categories: First generation (typical) and second generation (atypical). The main difference between the two types of antipsychotics is that the first generation drugs block dopamine and the second generation drugs block dopamine and also affect serotonin levels. Evidence suggests that some of the second generation drugs have milder movement-related side-effects than the first generation drugs.

Both categories of drugs work equally well overall, although no drug or type of drug works equally well for everyone who takes it. When the same drug is given to a group of people, one third of that group will find that it works well; another third will find that the drug helps only with some symptoms; and the final third will find that it does not help at all. For this reason, people may need to try different antipsychotics before finding the one that works best for them.

Most of these drugs are given in tablet form, some are liquids and others are given as injections. Some are available as long-lasting (depot) injections, which may be given anywhere from once a week to once a month.

Antipsychotics are often used in combination with other medications to treat other symptoms of mental health problems or to offset side-effects.

Most people who take antipsychotics over a longer term are now prescribed the second generation (also called atypical) drugs.

Second Generation (Atypical) Antipsychotics

Medications available in this class include risperidone (Risperdal)*, quetiapine (Seroquel), olanzapine (Zyprexa), ziprasidone (Zeldox), paliperidone (Invega), aripiprazole (Abilify) and clozapine (Clozaril). Clozapine is exceptional in that it often works even when other medications have failed; however, because it requires monitoring of white blood cell counts, it is not the first choice for treatment.

The second generation antipsychotics are usually the first choice for the treatment of schizophrenia. Although they may not be officially approved for these other uses, they are sometimes used in the treatment of mood and anxiety disorders, such as bipolar, post-traumatic stress and obsessive-compulsive disorders.

Some possible side-effects of this type of medication include dry mouth, dizziness, blurred vision and, rarely seizures. The Table 14.1 shows the side-effects of second generation antipsychotics and shows which drugs are most likely to least likely to have these effects.

| Table 14.1: Second generation antipsychotics ||
Side-effects of second generation antipsychotics	Drugs most likely to least likely to have these effects
Weight gain, diabetes	clozapine > olanzapine > quetiapine > risperidone > ziprasidone, aripiprazole
Movement effects (e.g. tremor, stiffness, agitation)	risperidone > olanzapine, quetiapine, ziprasidone, aripiprazole > clozapine
Sedation (e.g. sleepiness, low energy)	clozapine, olanzapine and quetiapine > risperidone, ziprasidone, aripiprazole
Decreased sex drive and function, missed periods, discharge from breasts	risperidone > olanzapine, quetiapine > clozapine, ziprasidone

First Generation (Typical) Antipsychotics

These older medications include chlorpromazine (once marketed as Largactil), flupenthixol (Fluanxol), fluphenazine (Modecate), haloperidol (Haldol), loxapine (Loxapac), perphenazine (Trilafon), pimozide (Orap), trifluoperazine (Stelazine), thiothixene (Navane) and zuclopenthixol (Clopixol).

Side-effects of this group of medications vary depending on the drug and may include drowsiness, agitation, dry mouth, constipation, blurred vision, emotional blunting, dizziness, stuffy nose, weight gain, breast tenderness, liquid discharge from breasts, missed periods, muscle stiffness or spasms.

Side-effects of Antipsychotics

Movement Effects

Tremors, muscle stiffness and tics can occur. The higher the dose, the more severe these effects. The risk of these effects may be lower with the second generation medications than with the older drugs. Other drugs (e.g. benztropine [Cogentin]) can be used to control the movement effects.

Dizziness

Feelings of dizziness may occur, especially when getting up from a sitting or lying position.

Weight Gain

Some of the second generation drugs are thought to affect people's sense of having had enough to eat. They can also be sedating. These two effects can result in weight gain, which can increase a person's risk of diabetes and heart disease.

Diabetes

Schizophrenia is a risk factor for diabetes. Antipsychotic drugs can increase this risk.

Agitation and Sedation

Some people feel "wired" and unable to stop moving when taking antipsychotics. This effect may be mistaken for a worsening of illness rather than a side-effect of the medication. These same drugs can also have the opposite effect, making people feel tired. Some people may feel either wired or tired, and some may feel both at the same time.

Tardive Dyskinesia

For every year that a person takes antipsychotic medication, there is a 5% chance of developing tardive dyskinesia (TD), a condition that causes people to have repetitive involuntary movements. The risk of TD is highest with the first generation antipsychotics, although it can occur with the second generation drugs. TD can worsen when you stop taking medication and can be permanent.

Neuroleptic Malignant Syndrome

This rare but serious complication is usually associated with the use of high doses of typical antipsychotics early in treatment. Signs include fever, muscle stiffness and delirium.

Controlling Side-effects

You can help to control possible side-effects on your own by:
- Getting regular exercise and eating a low-fat, low-sugar, high-fibre diet (e.g. bran, fruits and vegetables) to reduce the risk of diabetes and help prevent weight gain and constipation
- Using sugarless candy or gum, drinking water and brushing your teeth regularly to increase salivation and ease dry mouth
- Getting up slowly from a sitting or lying position to help prevent dizziness.

ANTIMANIC DRUGS

Antimanic agents are also called mood stabilizers.
For example, Lithium carbonate – 750 to 1000 mg/day
Carbomazapine 1.2 g/day
Valproric acid 750 mg/day
Indication: Mania, depression, bipolar mood disorder, schizoaffective disorder.

Action

It enhances the re-uptake or biogenic amines in the brain and lowers the level of amines in the body, resulting in decreased hyperactivity.

Contraindication: Cardiac vascular disease, severe renal disease, severe dehydration, pregnancy, lactation, hypothyroidism, history of seizure.

Side Effects

CNS—confusion, dizziness, weakness, headache, lethargy.
CVS—arrhythmias, hypotension, ECG changes.
Dermatology—drying and thinking of hair.
Endocrine—hypothyroidism.
GI tract—anorexia, nausea, vomiting, diarrhea, dry mouth, thirst.
GU tract—polyuric, glucosuria, oliguria.
Hematology—leukocylosis.

Interaction with Food

Increased dietary intake of Na will increase renal elimination of lithium.
Decreased dietary intake will cause retention of lithium and lead to toxicity.

Toxic Effects

Therapeutic blood lithium level 0.4 to 0.8 m and g/L is adequate
High range is 0.7 to 1.2 m and g/L
Toxicity level – more than 2 m and g/L
If it reach 3.5 m and g/L, it is life-threatening.

Toxic Symptoms

Ataxia, poor concentration of limb movement, slurred speech, confusion, coma, fits, death.

If the symptoms appear, lithium must be stopped at once and a high intake of fluid should be provided with extra NaCl to stimulate and increase osmotic diuretics. In severe cases, renal dialysis may be needed.

ANTIDEPRESSANT DRUGS

These are called as mood elevators or thymoleptics.

Indication

- Depression:
    - Depressive episode (MDP depression and endogenous depression)
    - Depressive episode with melancholia
    - Dysthymia
    - Reactive depression
    - Secondary depression (e.g. in hypothyroidism, Cushing's syndrome)
- Child psychiatric disorders: Enuresis, attention deficit disorders with hyperactivity, school phobia, somnambulism.
- Other psychiatric disorders: Panic attacks, OCD with or without depression, eating disorder, borderline personality disorder, post-traumatic stress disorders.
- Medical disorder: Chronic pain, migraine, peptic ulcer diseases.

Types of Antidepressant

1. **Tricyclic antidepressant (TCA)**
   For example, Imipramine—50–300 mg
   Trimipramine—50–300 mg
   Clomipramine—50–250 mg.

   Mechanism of Action
   Blocking the reuptake of norepinephrine and serotonin.
   It leads to increase the level of norepinephrine and serotonin at the synapse.

   Side Effects
   Autonomic: Dry mouth, urinary retention, constipation, postural hypotension, tachycardia, increased sweating.
   CVS: Tachycardia, hypotension, changes in ECG.
   Neurological: Tremors, in-coordination, headache, seizures.
   Others: Allergic skin rashes, mild jaundice, agranulocytosis.

2. **Monoamine oxidase inhibitors (MAOI)**
   For example, Isocarboxazid 20–60 mg
   Tranylcypromine 20–60 mg
   Monoamines: It includes nor epinephrine, epinephrine, dopamine and serotonin
   Monoamine oxidase (MAO): An enzyme that destroys monoamines
   MAOI: Drugs that prevent the destruction of monoamines by inhibiting the action of MAO.

3. **Selection serotonin reuptake inhibitions (SSRI)**
   Block the reuptake of serotonin.
   For example, sertraline—25–200 mg fluozatine, 20–80 mg.
   This is less side effect. It does not block muscarinic, and other receptors.

ANTI-ANXIETY DRUGS

Anti-anxiety drugs or anxiolytic drugs are minor tranquillizers.

Indication

- Management of anxiety disorder
- Acute alcoholic withdrawal
- Skeletal muscle spasms
- Convulsive disorders
- Preoperative sedation.

Classification of Anxiolytes

- Azaspirodecanadiones
  - Buspirone 100–400 mg
- Bendiazepines
  - Alprazolam 0.75–4 mg

- Diazepam 4–40 mg
- Lorazepam 2–6 mg.

Mechanism of Action

Anxiolytics depress subcritical level of CNS, particularly the limbic system and reticular formation. They may penetrate the effects of powerful inhibitory neurotransmitter gamma-aminobutyric acid (GABA) on the brain, thereby producing a calmative effect. All level of CNS depression can be affected from mild sedation to hypnosis to coma. But the drug buspirone does not depress the CNS, the drug is believed to produce the desired effects through interaction with serotonin dopamine and other neurotransmitter receptors.

One action of the benzodiazepine is to increase the GABA and help GABA open a chloride channel in and postsynaptic membrane of many neurons, thereby reducing the neurons excitability.

Increased effects of anxiolytics can occur when taken concomitantly with alcohol, barbiturates, narcotics, antipsychotics, antidepressants and antihistamine. Decreased effects can be noted with cigarette smoking and caffeine consumption.

Contraindication

- During or within 14 days of MAOI therapy
- Depressed or psychotic patients in the absence of anxiety
- First trimester of pregnancy and lactation
- Coma
- Acute alcoholic intoxication.

Side Effects

CNS—sedation, vertigo, weakness, ataxia, confusion
Ocular—blurred vision
Skin—rash, photosensitivity
GI—change in weight, dry mouth, constipation
CVS—tachycardia to cardiovascular collapse.

PSYCHOTHERAPY

Definition

Psychotherapy can be defined as "the treatment of emotional and/or related bodily problems by psychological means".

Psychotherapy is the development of a trusting relationship, which allows free communication and leads to understanding, integration and acceptance of self.

Objectives

- Finding out the cause of emotional problems
- Try to eliminate the cause

- Environmental manipulation to reduce the effect of distress
- Improve interpersonal relationship.

Types of Psychotherapy

Psychotherapies are classified according to:
a. Depth of probing in the unconscious mind
   i. Superficial or short-term or supportive psychotherapy
   ii. Deep or long-term or analytic psychotherapy
   iii. Educative psychotherapy.
b. Number of patients treated in any therapeutic sesstion
   i. Individual psychotherapy
   ii. Group psychotherapy
   iii. Family psychotherapy.
c. The purpose for which psychotherapy is given and the theoretical formulation used in psychotherapy
   i. Supportive psychotherapy: It provides support guidance, advice and re assurance
   ii. Re-educative psychotherapy: It attempts to teach the individual new patterns of behavior and social functioning.
   iii. Reconstructive psychotherapy: It aims to dismantle and rebuild a new personality.

Common Techniques Psychotherapy

- *Ventilation*: The process of allowing the release of bottled up emotions is called ventilation. The symptoms are the consequence of suppressed conflicts. This technique helps to express the suppressed emotions outwardly. Patient is allowed to talk whatever comes into his mind. The therapist notes the things which the client has expressed. He also note that patient knowingly avoid certain events. The patient is encouraged to talk about them more freely. Emotional distress should be avoided.
- *Abreaction*: It is a process of exploring the repressed emotions in a high degree. The person may sob during the therapy. The therapist facilitates the exploration without interruption. They should encourage the continuation by asking 'ok' then what happened?
- *Reassurance*: It is a supportive approach that any one can give. Our daily life itself indicates the effectiveness of one's reassurance in a critical situation. A re assurance like 'how silly it is, it will be solved. I am sure' can bring about marked change in distress.
- *Explanation*: It should be provided to remove misconceptions and to provide a proper understanding of the problem.
- *Suggestion*: It is a process by which symptoms relief is achieved through positive statements made with a degree of firmness and authority.

- *Persuasion*: It is a procedure by which the therapist urges the patient repeatedly to change his behavior or to try new methods of dealing with his problem.
- *Reinforcement:* Reinforcements or rewards are potent methods to enhance the desired behavior. They can be verbal or material in nature.
- *Recreation*: It helps to break monotony of work. It is especially required for subjects who have developed emotional problems as a result of having to perform monotonous and hard work.
- *Work as therapy*: Work is an important form of therapy for many types of emotional problems. When a person engages in work, his pre-occupation with his problems get lessened. It enhances his self-esteem, since he is not dependent on others.
- *Relaxation*: It is a technique especially useful for anxious individuals.

Unwanted Effects of Psychotherapy

- Patients may become excessively dependent on therapy or therapist.
- Intensive psychotherapy may be distressing to the patient
- Ineffective psychotherapy waste time and money, and damage patient's morale.

Contraindications

- Psychotic patients with severe behavior disturbances like excitement
- Organic psychosis
- Group psychotherapy is hysteria, hypochondriasis, etc.
- Patients who are unlikely to respond. For example, personality disorders.

BEHAVIOR THERAPY TECHNIQUES BASED ON CLASSICAL CONDITIONING

Introduction

- Behavior therapy involves changing the behavior of the patients to reduce the dysfunction and to improve the quality of life.
- The principles of behavior therapy are based on the early studies of classical conditioning by Pavlov (1927) and operant conditioning by Skinner (1938).
- Classical conditioning is the learning of involuntary responses by pairing a stimulus that normally causes a particular response with a new, neutral stimulus after enough parings, the new stimulus will also cause the response to occur.
- Through classical conditioning, the old and undesirable responses can be replaced by the desirable ones.
- There are several techniques that have been developed using this type of learning to treat the disorders such as phobias, obsessive compulsive disorder, and similar anxiety disorder.

Systematic Desensitization

- Developed by Wolpe and is based on the behavior principle of counter conditioning for assisting the individuals to overcome their fear of phobic stimulus.
- Systematic desensitization is a behavioral therapy technique where by a person overcomes the maladaptive anxiety elicited by a situation or an object by approaching the feared situation gradually, in a psychophysiological state that inhibits the anxiety.
- The technique of systematic desensitization in which a therapist guides the client through a series of steps meant to reduce the fear and anxiety.
- Systematic desensitization indicated in the cases of clearly identifiable anxiety provoking stimulus, such as:
  - Phobias
  - Obsessive compulsive disorder
  - Sexual disorders
  - Anxiety disorder.

Procedure

Systematic desensitization consist of three steps:
1. Relaxation training
2. Hierarchy construction
3. Desensitization of stimulus.

Relaxation Training

This is first step of systematic desensitization. Relaxation produces physiological effects opposite to those of anxiety.

The signs of relaxation are:
a. **Physiological signs:** Slow heart rate, increased peripheral blood flow and neuromuscular stability, pupil constriction, increased peripheral temperature, decreased oxygen consumption.
b. **Cognitive signs:** Altered state of consciousness, heightened concentration on single mental image.
c. **Behavior changes:** Lack of attention and concern for the environmental stimuli, no verbal interaction, no voluntary change in the position.

Techniques used for relaxation are:
a. Jacobson progressive muscle relaxation:
- Most often used relaxation training, developed by the psychiatrist Edmund Jacobson.
- In this client must learn to relax through deep muscle relaxation training.
- Patients relax major muscle group in a fixed order, beginning with the small muscle group of the feet and working cephal head or vice versa.

Procedure
  i. Make the patient in a comfortable position
  ii. Provide light or soft music/pleasant visual cues
  iii. Give a brief explanation about the progressive muscle relaxation
  iv. Instruct the client to tense each muscle group approximately for 10 seconds
  v. Explain the tension of the muscle and uncomfortable the body part feels
  vi. Ask the client to relax each muscle
  vii. Make client to feel the difference between both the situation.

b. Hypnosis
Some clinicians use hypnosis to facilitate the relaxation.

c. Mental imaginary
It is relaxation method in which patients are instructed to imagine the selves in a place associated with the pleasant relaxed memories.

Such images allow the patients to enter a relaxed state or experience the relaxation responses.

d. Meditation or yoga
Present days meditation and yoga are practiced and taught by the clinician to relax the patients, and it is an immerging trend in the relaxation therapy.

Hierarchy Construction

Hierarchy construction when constructing a hierarchy, clinicians determine all the conditions that elicit anxiety, and then patients create a hierarchy list consisting of 19 to 12 scenes in order of increasing the anxiety.

Example:
An example of a hierarchy of events associated with a fear of elevators as follows
a. Discuss riding an elevator with the therapist
b. Look at a picture of an elevator
c. Walk into the lobby of a building and see the elevators
d. Push the button for the elevator
e. Walk into the elevator with a trusted person, disembark before the door close
f. Walk into a elevator with a trusted person; allow the door to close; then open the door and walk out
g. Rise one floor with a trusted person, then walk down the stairs
h. Ride the elevator one floor with a trusted person and ride the elevator back down
i. Ride the elevator alone.

Desensitization

Desensitization of the stimulus in the final step, patients proceed systematically through the list from the least, to the most, anxiety provoking scene while in deeply relaxed state. Under the guidance of the therapist the client begins the

item on the list that causes minimal fear and looks at it, thinks about it, or actually confronts it, all while remaining in a relaxed state. The idea is that the phobic object or the situation is conditioned stimulus that the client has learned to fear because it was originally paired with a real fearful stimulus by paring the old conditioned stimulus with a new relaxation response that is compatible with the emotions and the physical arousal associated with the fear, the person's fear is reduced and relieved the person then proceeds to the next item on the hierarchy until the phobia is gone.

Adjunctive Use of the Drugs

Various drugs are used to hasten the relaxation. The advantage of the pharmacological desensitization are threat the preliminary training in the relaxation can be shortened, almost all patients can relax adequately. The drugs commonly used are, barbiturate sodium methohexital and diazepam.

Therapeutic Graded Exposure

Therapeutic graded exposure is similar to the systematic desensitization, except the relaxation training not involved and treatment is carried out in a real life context that is the individual must brought on contact with the warning stimulus to learn firsthand that no dangerous consequences will ensue exposure is graded according to the hierarchy, for example the patients afraid of cats might progress from looking at a picture of a cat holding one.

Aversion Therapy

Introduction

Aversion therapy is another way to use the classical conditioning is to reduce the frequency of the undesirable behavior, such as smoking or over eating, by teaching the client to pair an unpleasant stimulus that results in undesirable response.

Meaning

It is form of behavior therapy in which an undesirable behavior is paired with an aversive stimulus to reduce the frequency of the behavior.

Indication

- Alcohol abuse
- Paraphillias
- Homosexuality
- Tranvestism.

Types of Aversion Therapy

Overt Sensitization

It is a type of aversion therapy that produces unpleasant consequences for undesirable behavior. For example if an individual consumes alcohol while on

Antabuse therapy, symptoms of severe nausea, vomiting, dyspnea, palpitation and headache. Instead of euphoria feeling normally experienced from the alcohol, the individual receives a punishment that is intended to extinguish the unacceptable behavior.

Covert Sensitization

It relies on the individual produce symptoms rather than on medication. The technique is under clients control and can be used whenever and whenever it is required. The individual learns through mental imagery to visualize nauseating scenes and even to induce a mild feeling of nausea. It is most effective when paired with relaxation exercises that are performed instead of the undesirable behavior.

Preparation

Depending upon his/her customary practice, a therapist administering aversion therapy may establish a behavioral contract defining the treatment, objectives, expected outcome, and what will be required of the patient. The patient may be asked to keep a behavioral diary to establish a baseline measure of the behavior targeted for change. The patient undergoing this type of treatment should have enough information before hand to give full consent for the procedure. Patients with medical problems or who are otherwise vulnerable to potentially damaging physical side effects of the more intense aversive stimuli should consult their primary care doctor first.

Aftercare

Patients completing the initial phase of aversion therapy are often asked by the therapist to return periodically over the following six to twelve months or longer for booster sessions to prevent relapse.

Risks

Patients with cardiac, pulmonary, or gastrointestinal problems may experience a worsening of their symptoms, depending upon the characteristics and strength of the aversive stimuli. Some therapists have reported that patients undergoing aversion therapy, especially treatment that uses powerful chemical or pharmacological aversive stimuli, have become negative and aggressive.

Examples

- Someone who wants to stop smoking might go to the therapist who uses a rapid smoking techniques, in which the client is allowed to smoke but must take the puff on the cigarette every five or six seconds. As nicotine is a poison, such rapid smoking produces nausea and dizziness, both unpleasant responses.
- Cigarette including the act of putting into the mouth, lighting up (CS) which leads to a pleasurable stimulation response (CR), then rapid smoking (US) which leads to nausea and dizziness (UR). Repeated practice lead to the unconditioned response (UR) to a conditioned response (CR).

- Use of a drug called disulfiram to treat the alcoholism is another example for the aversion therapy. This medicine is properly prescribed and monitored results in several aversive reactions when combined with the alcohol. The person may experience nausea, vomiting and anxiety, and even more serious symptoms making this drug an effective deterrent for drinking for people who are unable to quit by other means.

Flooding

Introduction

Flooding was invented by a psychologist named Thomas Stampfl. Flooding is an effective form of treatment for phobias amongst other psychopathologies. It works on the behaviorist principles of classical conditioning.

Meaning

It is behavior therapy technique in which the person is rapidly and intensely exposed to the fear provoking situation or object and prevented from making the usual avoidance or escape response.

Indication

- Phobias
- Post-traumatic stress disorder
- Obsessive compulsive disorder.

Procedure

Flooding is based on the premise that escaping from an anxiety provoking reinforces the anxiety through conditioning client is prevented from the conditioned avoidance of the behavior by not allowing the patient to escape the situation. No relaxation therapy is used and patient experiences fear. Which gradually subsides after some time. The success of the procedure depends on having the patients remain in the fear generating situation until they are calm and feel a sense of mastery.

Advantage of Classical Conditioning Techniques

- Short duration of therapy
- Easy to train the clients
- Cot effective
- Duration of treatment is usually 6–8 weeks.

COGNITIVE BEHAVIOR THERAPY (CBT)

Introduction

- CBT is a psychotherapeutic approach that aims to solve problems concerning dysfunctional emotions, behaviors and cognitions through a goal-oriented, systematic procedure.

- CBT combines the cognitive therapy developed by Aron Beck and behavior therapy techniques.
- Thoughts cause feelings and behaviors
- Emphasis placed on current behavior.
- CBT is a collaborative effort between the therapist and the client.
  - Client role—define goals, express concerns, learn and implement learning
  - Therapist role—help client define goals, listen, teach, encourage.
- Based on "rational thought"—fact not assumptions.
- CBT is structured and directive. Based on notion that maladaptive behaviors are the result of skill deficits.
- Homework is a central feature of CBT.
- Cognitive therapies do not appear to work as well with those who are cognitively impaired.

Definition

- Focused form of psychotherapy based on a model suggesting that psychiatric/psychological disorders involve dysfunctional thinking
- The way an individual feels and behaves in influenced by the way she/he structures his experiences.
- Modifying dysfunctional thinking provides improvements in symptoms and modifying dysfunctional beliefs that underlie dysfunctional thinking leads to more durable improvement.

Indications

Cognitive therapy was originally developed for use in the treatment of depression.
- Personality disoders
- Seasonal affective disorders
- Generalized anxiety disorders
- Obsessive-compulsive disorders
- Mood disorders-depression.

Major Concepts and Procedure

The General Cognitive Model

Situation
↓
Automatic thoughts and images
↓
Reaction (emotional, behavior and physiological)

The Cognitive Triad

- Negative view of the self (e.g. I am unlovable, ineffective)
- Negative view of the future (e.g. nothing will work out)
- Negative view of the world (e.g. world is hostile)

Automatic Thoughts

- Negative thoughts about yourself, your world, or your future
- Examples of automatic thoughts:
  - Catastrophizing—extreme consequences of events
  - All or nothing—seeing things in black and white—no grey areas
  - Emotional reasoning—if I feel it, it must be true.

Helplessness

- I am inadequate, ineffective, incompetent, can not cope
- I am powerless, out of control, trapped
- I am vulnerable, likely to be hurt, weak, needy
- I am inferior, a failure, a lower, not good enough, defective, do not measure up.

Hopelessness

- I am unlikable, unwanted, will be rejected or abandoned, always be alone
- I am undesirable, unattractive, ugly, boring, have nothing to offer
- I am different, defective, not good enough to be loved by other, a nerd

The Cognitive Model

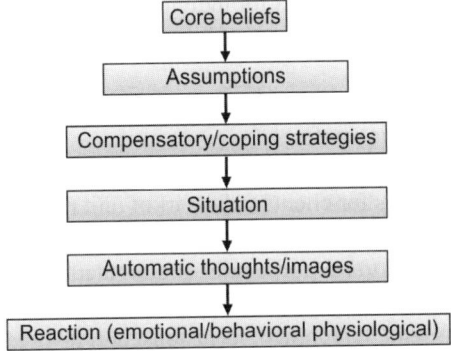

The Basic Goals of CBT

- To challenge the thoughts about a particular situation by identifying the cognitive traps
- To help the patient to identify less threatening alternatives
- To test out these alternatives in the real world
- To challenge the assumptions that lead to the automatic thoughts

The Basic Tenets of CBT

- Cognitive specificity
- Socratic dialogue
- Collaborative empiricism.

MILIEU THERAPY

Meaning

The word milieu is French for "middle". The English translation of the word is surroundings or environment. Milieu therapy is the scientific planning of an environment for therapeutic purposes.

Definition

A scientific structuring of the environment in order to effect behavioral changes and to improve the psychological health and functioning of the individual (Skinner, 1979).

Goals of Milieu Therapy

- Manipulate the environment, so that all aspects of client's hospital experience are considered therapeutic
- Client is expected to learn adaptive coping, interaction and relationship skills that can be generalized to other aspects of his or her life
- Achieving client autonomy.

Principles of Milieu Therapy

- To promote a fundamental respect for individuals (both clients and staff)
- To use opportunities for communication between client and staff for maximum therapeutic benefit
- To encourage clients to act at a level equal to their ability and to enhance their self-esteem (autonomy is reinforced)
- To promote socialization
- To provide opportunities for clients to be part of unit management
- Individuals are held responsible for own actions
- Peer pressure is utilized to reinforce rules and regulations
- Team approach is used
- Group discussions and temporary seclusions are favored approaches for acting out behavior
- The nurses function is to act in ways that consistently promote these goals.

Characteristics of Milieu Therapy

The concept of milieu therapy developed from a desire to counteract the negative, regressive effects of institutionalization: Reduced ability to think and act independently, an adoption of institutional values and attitudes, and loss of commitments in the outside world.

Several strategies have been developed to counter these negative effects. They include:
- Distribution of power
- Open communication

- Structured interactions
- Work-related activities
- Community and family involvement in the treatment process
- Adaptation of the environment to meet developmental needs.

Distribution of Power

- The milieu therapy approach involves "flattening" the control hierarchy so all participants have a voice in decision making. This process may include the whole population of the treatment unit, or a governing council may take the final decisions based on input from various smaller groups of clients and staff members.
- The ultimate goal of any treatment program is client autonomy. This may be achieved through a stepwise progression through a number of treatment programs or by gradually increasing independence within a given program. Consciously incorporating a plan for increasing independence is a means to achieve client autonomy.

Open Communication

- Although the importance of open communication has been widely recognized in literature, it is still not a reality in many settings. One reason for this may be the insecurity of persons in the authority. Open communication requires risk taking. Questioning and criticism may be threatening, whereas there is little to risk if no feedback is allowed. Cultural norms, personal defenses and established communication patterns may block the communications.
- In the therapeutic milieu, treatment decisions are often made by the clients themselves, who therefore need information to make effective decision. It is not necessary to communicate personal information but clients and staff need to be aware of individual treatment goals to ensure everyone is working towards the same goal. In this atmosphere, exclusive confidentiality is replaced by mutual trust, honesty and open communication.

Structured Interactions

- KA Menninger pioneered the concept of structured interaction patterns in the form of attitude therapy. An advantage of the structured interaction approach is that all staff members approach the client in a consistent manner, acknowledging specific diagnostic areas, thereby shortening treatment time.
- The difficulty with this approach is that once a diagnosis is made and an attitude prescribed there is little flexibility in the interaction pattern. Day-to-day fluctuations in the client's condition may not be accounted for, and some staff members sometimes seem stilted in their response to clients.

Work-related Activities

- The focus of these activities is on benefits to the client rather than to the agency. Work under realistic circumstances and for appropriate rewards is

probably the best central activity for all clients. Several factors contribute to effective work therapy programs.
- First, clients need to choose the type of work they wish to perform
- Second, work activities should be geared toward developing skills that will be useful in actual job situations. The current trend is to place clients on the job and provide funds for staff support in the work environment.
- Third, a variety of activities provides the opportunity to test different areas for future job interests.

Community and Family Involvement

- As a result of more effective medications and humane treatment philosophies, community mental health centers emerged. Hospitalization is considered desirable only for acute illnesses. For easy accessibility, mental health centers are placed conveniently within a neighborhood.
- According to milieu therapy approach, clients are kept in their usual environment, for example, a day treatment center or halfway house, and continue most of their routine activities while receiving treatment. If one family member is hospitalized, an attempt is made to continue family involvement. This is an effective way to improve family interaction and minimize the isolation resulting from hospitalizing one family member.

Adaptation of the Environment to Meet the Developmental Needs

- To develop his full potential an individual must have an environment adapted to his current needs. Adapting the environment to meet these multiple needs is challenging due to the extension of milieu therapy to all age groups and the inclusion of family members with individuals of varying ages within the treatment milieu.
- Clients who are regressed or who are overwhelmed need more structure and support; other clients benefit from a program that promotes autonomy and responsibility. A program that provides stepwise increase in responsibility would be an effective solution.

Programs within the milieu

1. **Client Government:**
- Structured meeting
- Clients have inputs into all unit activities
- May make decisions related to privileges for other clients
- Discussion of the problems of everyday living
- Usually meets once per week.
2. **Work-related activities:**
- Work therapy
- Monetary reward
- Client should choose the type of work
- Offer a variety of activities.

Advantages and Disadvantages of Milieu Therapy

Advantages

- Milieu therapy creates a different type of attitude and behavior in the patient because the environment is like home.
- Instead of adopting a sick role, the patient makes decisions in the ward management and cares for other patients. In other words, he becomes less dependent and passive.
- The patient learns to adopt a behavior which is acceptable in the therapeutic environment like learns to control hostility.
- The patient learns to make decisions which improves his self-confidence.
- Milieu includes safe physical surroundings, all the treatment team members, and other clients, which is supported by clear and consistently maintained limits and behavioral expectations.
- A therapeutic milieu is a safe space, a non-punitive atmosphere, which minimize the environmental stress and provides a chance for rest and nurturance of self, a time to focus on the developments of strengths, and an opportunity to learn to identify alternatives or solutions to problems and to learn about the psychodynamics of those problems.
- Patient develops harmonious relationships with other members of the community.
- Develops leadership skills.
- Becomes socio centric.
- Learns to live and think collectively with the members of the community.

Disadvantages

- Role blurring between staff and patient.
- Group responsibility can easily become nobody's responsibility.
- Individual needs and concerns may not be met.
- Patient may find the transition to community difficult.
- Milieu therapy is limited to only hospitalized patients.
- Conflict resolution is needed as part of the staff's skills.
- Low client-to-staff ratio.
- Requires continuous open communication among all staff and clients.

THERAPEUTIC COMMUNITY

Definition

"A therapeutic community is a drug-free environment in which people with addictive (and other) problems live together in an organized and structured way in order to promote change and make possible a drug-free life in the outside society. The therapeutic community forms a miniature society in which residents, and staff in the role of facilitators, fulfill distinctive roles and adhere to clear rules, all designed to promote the transitional process of the residents" (Ottenberg 1993).

Stuart and Sundeen defined therapeutic community as "a therapy in which patient's social environment would be used to provide a therapeutic experience for the patient by involving him as an active participant in his own care and the daily problems of his community".

Objectives

- To use patient's social environment to provide a therapeutic experience for him
- To enable the patient to be an active participant in his own care and become involved in daily activities of his own community
- To help patient to solve problems, plan activities and to develop the necessary rules and regulations for the community
- To increase their independence and gain control over many of their own personal activities
- To enable the patient to become aware of how their behavior affects others.

Elements of Therapeutic Community

- Free communication
- Shared responsibility
- Active participation
- Involvement in decision making
- Understanding of the roles, responsibilities, limitations and authorities.

Components of Therapeutic Community

a. Daily community meetings

- These meetings are composed of 60–90 patients. All levels of unit staff are involved, including administrative personnel. Acute patients are not involved in the meetings
- Meetings should be held regularly for 60 minutes
- Discussion should focus mainly on day-to-day life in the unit
- During discussion patients feelings and behaviors are examined by other members
- Frank discussion are encouraged, these may take place with much out poring of emotions and anger.

b. Patient Government or Ward Council

- The purpose of patient government is to deal with practical unit details such as house-keeping functions, activity planning and privileges
- A group of 5–6 patients will have specific responsibilities, such as house-keeping, physical exercise, personal hygiene, meal distribution, a group to observe suicidal patients. Staff members should be always available
- All decisions should be feedback to the community through the community meetings.

c. **Staff meetings or review**
- A staff meeting should be held following each community meeting (patients are excluded and only staff are present). In this meeting the staff would examine their own responses, expectations and prejudice.

d. **Living and learning opportunities**
- Learning opportunities are provided within the social milieu, which should provide realistic learning experiences for the patients.

Length of Treatment in a Therapeutic Community

In general, individuals progress through drug addiction treatment at varying speeds, so there is no predetermined length of treatment. Those who complete treatment achieve the best outcomes, but even those who drop out may receive some benefit. Good outcomes from therapeutic community (TC) treatment are strongly related to treatment duration, which likely reflects benefits derived from the underlying treatment process. Individuals who complete at least 90 days of treatment in a TC have significantly better outcomes on average than those who stay for shorter periods.

Traditionally, stays in TCs have varied from 18 to 24 months. Recently, however, funding restrictions have forced many TCs to significantly reduce stays to 12 months or less and/or develop alternatives to the traditional residential model. For individuals with many serious problems (e.g. multiple drug addictions, criminal involvement, mental health disorders, and low employment), research again suggests that outcomes were better for those who received TC treatment for 90 days or more.

In the TC, the level of treatment engagement and participation is related to retention and outcomes. Treatment factors associated with increased retention include having a good relationship with one's counselor, being satisfied with the treatment, and attending education classes. Important attributes linked to treatment retention include self-esteem, attitudes and beliefs about oneself and one's future, and readiness and motivation for treatment. Retention can be improved through interventions to address these areas.

Advantages of Therapeutic Community

- Patient develops harmonious relationships with other members of the community
- Gains self-confidence
- Develops leadership skills
- Learns to understand and solve problems of self and others
- Becomes socio-centric
- Learns to live and think collectively with the members of the community
- It provides opportunity to participate in the formulation of hospital rules and regulations that affect patient's personal liberties like bedtime, meal time, weekend permission, control of radio or TV, social activities, late night privileges.

Disadvantages of Therapeutic Community

- Role blurring between staff and patient
- Group responsibility can easily become nobody's responsibility
- Individual needs and concerns may not be met
- Patient find the transition to community difficult.

FAMILY THERAPY

Family therapy was started by Bateson in 1956 and was well developed by Nathan Ackerman group in 1958.

Family therapy is an essential interventions in a family system to change the family. The family is the unit which is being treated for better interactions among each other.

Aims

- Helping the family members clarify and express their feelings towards one another
- To remove transitional-generational gap
- To establish good communication pattern
- To develop greater mutual understanding.

Indications

- Marital problem.
- Child mental health problems
- Adjustment disorder
- Alcoholism and drug dependence
- Attempted suicide.

Contraindications

- Lack of adequately trained therapist
- Poor motivation
- Fixed character pathology, e.g. lying, physical violence.

Types

1. Structural family therapy: In a structured family therapy, change the origin of the family in such a way that the family members behave more positively and supportively towards each other.
2. Systemic family therapy: This is based on the concept that families are systems where:
    i. Individual are not independent
    ii. In the pursuit of homeostasis changes are often focused on one individual when presents as the problem.

3. Strategic family therapy: It is a problem based therapy, where although understanding the meaning of the problem is important. It is not the basis for interventions.

MARITAL THERAPY (COUPLES THERAPY)

Martial therapy is helpful to improve marital relationship. Therapist tries to find out the problems between partners can share their perceptions about their relationship. Therapist can help to find out solutions for the couples problems.

OCCUPATIONAL THERAPY (OT)

Definition

Occupation therapy defined as a profession concerned with promoting health and well being through occupation.

Goal

- Increasing functioning and independence
- Maintaining or increasing skills
- Adapting environment to meet the unique needs of an individuals
- To provide intervention.

Indications

- Traumatic injuries (brain or spiral cord)
- Learning problem
- Autism
- Pervasive developmental disorder
- Mental health or behavioral problems
- Developmental delays.

Therapeutic Activities

These are purposeful activities including arts, crafts, recreation, sports, leisure, self-care, home management and work activities which help to:
- Develop or maintain strength, endurance and range of motion
- Provide the use of voluntary, automatic movements in goal direction tasks
- Exercise effected parts of the body
- Identify vocation potential and work training
- Improve sensation, perception and cognition
- Develop social skills.

Types of Occupational Therapy

Any vocation which earns ones livelihood can be used. Therapies commonly used in hospital as a rehabilitation therapy are pottery therapy, carpentry, candle making, basketing, mat weaving, tailoring, craft, etc.

Process of Intervention

It consists of following stages:
1. Initial evaluation of what patient can do and cannot do
2. Development of immediate and long-term goals by patient and therapist together
3. Develop therapy plan with planned intervention
4. Implement the plan
5. Call for review meetings with patient and all the staff involved in treatment
6. When immediate goals have been achieved set further goals and alter the treatment program
7. Highlight the monitoring when the patient is ready to discontinue treatment.

Settings

Occupational therapy is provided in psychiatric units, psychosocial and physical rehabilitation centers, sheltered work-shops or clinics, special schools for physically and mentally handicapped, integrated schools, community group homes, community mental health centers, day care centers, industrial health unit, halfway homes and in deaddiction centers.

MUSIC THERAPY

Music therapy is the functional application music toward the attainment of specific therapeutic goals.

Goal

- To reduce psychophysiological stress, pain and anxiety
- It leads to slower heart rate, respiratory rate and BP.

Effects of Music Therapy

- Soothing music can be used to achieve an alpha wave brain state which initiates a state of relaxed awareness.
- Soothing music with a flowing, lyrical, melody, single, harmony and soft tone helps to stimulate the relaxation response.
- It facilitates emotional homeostasis.
- Music therapy influences the physiological variables like BP, HR, respiratory, EEG measurements and body temperature.
- Alleviates pain, anxiety, nausea, fatigue and depression.
- Lowers apical heart rate.
- Enhances sleep.
- Music can encourage socialization, self-expression, communication and motor development.

DANCE/MOVEMENT THERAPY

It is a psychotherapeutic use of movement and dance for emotional, cognitive, social, behavioral and physical condition.

It strengthens the body/mind connection through body movements to improve both mental and physical welling of individuals.

Indication

Emotionally disturbed, depression and suicidal, MR, substance abusers, visually and hearing impaired, psychotics, autistic, cancer, anorexia and bulimia, heart disease, diabetes, AIDS, arthritis.

Advantages

- Helps to develop body awareness
- Facilitates empression of feelings
- Improve interaction and communication
- Increased sense of self-confidence.

Principles of Dance Movement Therapy

It is based upon the idea that the body and mind are inseparable
- Body and mind interact, so that a change in movement will affect total functioning
- Movement reflects personality
- The therapeutic relationship is medicated at least to some extent nonverbally.

PSYCHODRAMA

Psychodrama is a special form of group therapy which provides the patient with an additional opportunity to gain self-insight. It uses structured directed dramatizations of a patient's emotional problems and experiences.

Members are encourage to act out immediate or past life situation, conflicts or problems.

Aims

To develop greater awareness to patient about his thoughts, feelings and actions and of how they affect others.

Indications

Marital discord, alcoholics.

Advantages

- It helps the patient to define his problem clearly
- To explore the patient's adaptive and maladaptive coping response to his problem.
- To identify misperceptions, unrealistic goals and distortions of reality.

RECREATIONAL THERAPY

Recreation is a form of activity therapy used in most psychiatric setting.

Classification of Recreational Activities

The various forms of play or activity used in recreational therapy are:
1. Motor forms:
   These can be further divided into fundamental and accessory, based on whether the motor element is the main purpose of the activity or merely incidental to it. Among the fundamental forms are such games as hockey and football. While the accessory forms are exemplified by play-activity and dancing.
2. The sensory forms may be either visual, e.g. looking at motion picture, play etc. or auditory such as listening to a concert.
3. The intellectual forms include such activities as reading, debating, etc.
   In recreational therapy recreation is regarded in its every sphere, and the following shows the wide range in which it is used:
   - Goal games, e.g. hide and seek
   - Team games, e.g. hockey and football
   - Country sports, e.g. shooting, fishing
   - Combats, e.g. wrestling, boring
   - Curiosity play, e.g. crossword puzzles
   - Creative play, e.g. play-acting
   - Vicarious play, e.g. viewing at motion pictures
   - Imitative play, e.g. follow the leader in fold dancing
   - Social play, e.g. party games
   - Aesthetic play, e.g. painting and clay modeling
   - Acquisition play, e.g. collecting antiques or stamps.

Aims
- To train memory and concentration
- To re-educate mentally, psychically and socially
- To give a sense of responsibility, e.g. by giving an opportunity to organize or lead a game
- To stimulate interest
- To stimulate or recreate self-confidence
- To arouse and develop attention
- To give an opportunity for self-expression
- To replace unhealthy trends by healthy one
- To substitute encouragement for discouragement
- To improve the appetite
- To improve the circulation
- To improve respiration
- To strengthen the tone of the muscles
- To develop a sense of rhythm
- To develop a good posture.

LIGHT THERAPY

Light therapy or phototherapy consists of emposing a patient to artificial therapeutic lighting about 5 to 20 times brighter than indoor lighting. Patients usually sit, with eyes open about 3 feet away from and at eye level with a set of broad spectrum fluorescent bulbs designed to produce the intensity and color composition of outdoor daylight.

The timing and dosage of the light vary from person to person. Most literature indicates that light treatment administrated in the morning is more effective.

Light therapy appears to have important positive effects. Treatment is rapid and can be repeated. Most patients feel relief after 3 to 5 days, and they relapse equally rapidly after light treatment is stopped.

Indications: Seasonal affective disorder (SAD), non-seasonal depression, bulimia nervosa, premenstrual syndrome.

Mechanism of Action

The therapeutic effect appears to be mediated primarily by the eyes, not the skin. Ongoing studies of the mechanism of light therapy are exploring the eye itself, the way in which the eyes send message to the brain, and the role of brain neurotransmitter systems such as serotonin and dopamine. It also appears that certain people may have a neurochemical vulnerability, possibly inherited, that causes them to develop SAD in the absence of adequate exposure to environmental light.

Side Effects

The common side effects are eyestrain, headache, irritability, insomnia, nausea and dryness of the eyes, nasal passages and sinuses.

ELECTROCONVULSIVE THERAPY

Introduction

- ECT is a physical therapy in which with the help of electrodes, electrical current is passed to the brain to produce generalized seizures.
- Modified electroconvulsive therapy (ECT) is a controlled medical procedure in which a seizure is induced in an anesthetized patient to produce a therapeutic effect. (Kavanagh and McLoughlin, 2009).
- Electroconvulsive therapy (ECT) is a highly technical procedure requiring a team that consists of an anesthetist, a psychiatrist, psychiatric nurses, and recovery nurses.
- Psychiatric nurses have an important role in caring patients who receive ECT.

Indications

ECT is the most acutely effective treatment available for affective disorders and is more effective than antidepressant drugs. (Kavanagh and McLoughlin, 2009).

ECT may be considered as a *primary treatment (or first-line treatment)* for persons exhibiting syndromes such as: Severe major depression, acute mania, mood disorders with psychotic features, and catatonia.
- Severe depression
- Acute mania
- Mood disorders with psychotic features
- Intolerance to side effects of medication or other treatments
- Deterioration in condition, or appearance of suicidality or pronounced lethargy
- Acute catatonia.

Contraindications

Contraindications to ECT include brain tumors, space-occupying lesions, and other brain diseases that cause increased intracranial pressure.

Nursing Care in ECT

Electroconvulsive therapy is treated like a minor surgical procedure that requires preoperative preparation and postoperative care. (Arkan B, Ustün B, 2008). There are four components of nursing care in ECT:
- Providing educational and emotional support
- Pretreatment planning and assessment
- Preparing and monitoring the patient during the actual procedure
- Post-treatment care and evaluation.

Providing Educational and Emotional Support

- Explain the procedure to the patient
- Obtain an informed consent from the patient and the carer
- Respond to patient's concerns and feelings
- Educate the patient concerning the procedure and explain to the patient the necessary tasks associated with ECT
- Initiate education interventions based on knowledge deficits.

Pretreatment Nursing Care

- Preparation of treatment suite for the ECT procedure
- An adjustable height stretcher trolley
- Complete the pretreatment checklist
- The patient's identity is checked and the patient wears an identity bracelet
- Ensure safekeeping of the patient's valuables
- NPO for minimum 4 hours before treatment to prevent possible aspiration during anesthesia
- The patient's hair should be clean and dry to allow for electrode contact
- Hairpins, bracelets, body piercing should be removed to avoid burns
- The patient should be encouraged to pass urine before the treatment to avoid incontinence during the procedure

- Prostheses, dentures, glasses, hearing aids, contact lenses, should be removed
- Minimize anxiety through anxiety management techniques, ensuring short waiting time and offering reassurance and support
- Standard practices should be practiced regarding general anesthesia care.

Nursing Care during ECT Procedure

- Transfer the patient on a trolley from the waiting room to the ECT room on a well padded bed and placed in a comfortable dorsal position or supine position. A small pillow is placed under the lumber curve.
- Apply ECG electrodes, BP cuff, and pulse oximetry sensor (not on same extremity as BP cuff).
- Give a short acting anesthetic agent. Thiopental. 0.25–0.5 mg, IV and Secoline (succinyl choline) 30–50 mg. The dose of drug may vary from patient to patient.
- Prepare EEG electrodes, per-treatment specifications.
- Prepare scalp and stimulus ECT electrodes (unilateral vs. bilateral) and apply paste to electrodes.
- Support the shoulder and arms of the patient. Restraint the thigh with the help of a sheet.
- Hyperextension of the head with support to the chin.
- Administer oxygen
- Apply jelly to the electrodes
- Make the observations of the convulsions.
- The presence of initial tonic stage which lasts for 10–15 seconds followed by clonic stage which lasts for 25–30 seconds then there is a phase of muscular relaxation with stertorus respiration, i.e. flaccid stage.
- Do suction immediately
- Restore respiration by giving O_2 if necessassry.

Post-ECT Care

- Observe and record the vital parameters
- Place the patient on side-lying position, clean the secretions
- Transfer the patient from recovery room, record vital signs every 15 minutes for 30 minutes and once in every 30 minutes till the patient recover to the normal stage
- Allow the patient to sleep for 30 minutes to 1 hour
- Reassure the client and reorient to the ward
- Allow the patient to have tea or any drinks
- Record the procedure.

Equipment for ECT

- Treatment devices and supplies, including electrode paste and gel, gauze pads, saline, electroencephalogram electrodes and chart paper.
- Monitoring equipments including ECG and EEG electrodes

- BP cuffs, peripheral nerve stimulator and pulse oxymeter
- Stethoscope
- Reflex hammer
- Intravenous and venipuncture supplies
- Stretchers with firm mattress with side rails with the capacity of raising the head and foot end
- Bite blocks
- Suction device
- Ventilation equipment, including tubing, masks, Ambu bag, oral airways, intubations equipments with an oxygen delivery system capable of providing positive- pressure oxygen
- Emergency and other medications as recommended by the anesthesia staff
- Miscellaneous medications not supplied by anesthesia staff for medical management during ECT such as midazolam, diazepam, thiopental sodium, glycopyrolate, succinyl choline, etc.

ALTERNATIVE APPROACHES TO MENTAL HEALTH TREATMENT

Culturally Based Healing Arts

Traditional oriental medicine (such as *acupuncture*, shiatsu, and reiki), Indian systems of health care (such as Ayurveda and Yoga), and Native American healing practices (such as the Sweat Lodge and Talking Circles) all incorporate the beliefs that:
- Wellness is a state of balance between the spiritual, physical, and mental/emotional "selves."
- An imbalance of forces within the body is the cause of illness.
- Herbal/natural remedies, combined with sound nutrition, exercise, and meditation/prayer, will correct this imbalance.

Acupuncture: The Chinese practice of inserting needles into the body at specific points manipulates the body's flow of energy to balance the endocrine system. This manipulation regulates functions such as heart rate, body temperature, and respiration, as well as sleep patterns and emotional changes. Acupuncture has been used in clinics to assist people with substance abuse disorders through detoxification; to relieve stress and anxiety; to treat attention deficit and hyperactivity disorder in children; to reduce symptoms of depression; and to help people with physical ailments.

Ayurveda: Ayurvedic medicine is described as "knowledge of how to live." It incorporates an individualized regimen—such as diet, meditation, herbal preparations, or other techniques—to treat a variety of conditions, including depression, to facilitate lifestyle changes, and to teach people how to release stress and tension through yoga or transcendental meditation.

Yoga/meditation: Practitioners of this ancient Indian system of health care use breathing exercises, posture, stretches, and meditation to balance the body's

energy centers. Yoga is used in combination with other treatment for depression, anxiety, and stress-related disorders.

Native American traditional practices: Ceremonial dances, chants, and cleansing rituals are part of Indian Health Service Programs to heal depression, stress, trauma (including those related to physical and sexual abuse), and substance abuse.

Cuentos: Based on folktales, this form of therapy originated in Puerto Rico. The stories used contain healing themes and models of behavior such as self-transformation and endurance through adversity. Cuentos is used primarily to help Hispanic children recover from depression and other mental health problems related to leaving one's homeland and living in a foreign culture.

Relaxation and Stress Reduction Techniques

Biofeedback: Learning to control muscle tension and "involuntary" body functioning, such as heart rate and skin temperature, can be a path to mastering one's fears. It is used in combination with, or as an alternative to, medication to treat disorders such as anxiety, panic, and phobias. For example, a person can learn to "retrain" his or her breathing habits in stressful situations to induce relaxation and decrease hyperventilation. Some preliminary research indicates it may offer an additional tool for treating schizophrenia and depression.

Guided imagery or visualization: This process involves going into a state of deep relaxation and creating a mental image of recovery and wellness. Physicians, nurses, and mental health providers occasionally use this approach to treat alcohol and drug addictions, depression, panic disorders, phobias, and stress.

Massage therapy: The underlying principle of this approach is that rubbing, kneading, brushing, and tapping a person's muscles can help release tension and pent emotions. It has been used to treat trauma-related depression and stress. A highly unregulated industry, certification for massage therapy varies widely from State to State. Some States have strict guidelines, while others have none.

Technology-based Applications

The boom in electronic tools at home and in the office makes access to mental health information just a telephone call or a "mouse click" away. Technology is also making treatment more widely available in once-isolated areas.

Telemedicine: Plugging into video and computer technology is a relatively new innovation in health care. It allows both consumers and providers in remote or rural areas to gain access to mental health or specialty expertise. Telemedicine can enable consulting providers to speak to and observe patients directly. It also can be used in education and training programs for generalist clinicians.

Telephone counseling: Active listening skills are a hallmark of telephone counselors. These also provide information and referral to interested callers. For

many people telephone counseling often is a first step to receiving in-depth mental health care. Research shows that such counseling from specially trained mental health providers reaches many people who otherwise might not get the help they need. Before calling, be sure to check the telephone number for service fees; a 900 area code means you will be billed for the call, an 800 or 888 area code means the call is toll-free.

Electronic communications: Technologies such as the internet, bulletin boards, and electronic mail lists provide access directly to consumers and the public on a wide range of information. On-line consumer groups can exchange information, experiences, and views on mental health, treatment systems, alternative medicine, and other related topics.

Radio psychiatry: Another relative newcomer to therapy, radio psychiatry was first introduced in the United States in 1976. Radio psychiatrists and psychologists provide advice, information, and referrals in response to a variety of mental health questions from callers. The American Psychiatric Association and the American Psychological Association have issued ethical guidelines for the role of psychiatrists and psychologists on radio shows.

Chapter 15

Community Mental Health

Community mental health defined as the process of involving in raising the level of mental health among people in a community and reducing the number of those suffering from mental disorder.

The basis model of community mental health was defined by Gerald Caplan in 1967. The predominant characteristics of community psychiatry are:
- Responsibility to a population for mental health care delivery
- Treatment close to the patient in community based centers
- Provision of comprehensive services
- Multi-disciplinary team approach
- Providing continuity of case
- Emphasis on prevention as well as treatment
- Avoidance of unnecessary hospitalization.

NATIONAL MENTAL HEALTH PROGRAM

Psychiatric symptoms are common in general population in both sides of the globe. These symptoms—worry, tiredness, and sleepless nights affect more than half of the adults at some time, while as many as one person in seven experiences some form of diagnosable neurotic disorder.

Burden of Disease

The World Bank report (1993) revealed that the Disability Adjusted Life Year (DALY) loss due to neuropsychiatric disorder is much higher than diarrhea, malaria, worm infestations and tuberculosis if taken individually. According to the estimates DALYs loss due to mental disorders are expected to represent 15% of the global burden of diseases by 2020.

During the last two decades, many epidemiological studies have been conducted in India, which show that the prevalence of major psychiatric disorder is about the same all over the world. The prevalence reported from these studies range from the population of 18 to 207 per 1000 with the median 65.4 per 1000 and at any given time, about 2–3 % of the population, suffer from seriously, incapacitating mental disorders or epilepsy. Most of these patients live in rural areas remote from any modern mental health facilities. A large number of adult patients (10.4–53%) coming to the general OPD are diagnosed mentally ill. However, these patients are usually missed because either medical officer or general practitioner at the primary health care unit does not asked detailed mental health history. Due to

the under-diagnosis of these patients, unnecessary investigations and treatments are offered which heavily cost to the health providers.

Program

The Government of India has launched the National Mental Health Program (NMHP) in 1982, keeping in view the heavy burden of mental illness in the community, and the absolute inadequacy of mental health care infrastructure in the country to deal with it.

Aims

1. Prevention and treatment of mental and neurological disorders and their associated disabilities.
2. Use of mental health technology to improve general health services.
3. Application of mental health principles in total national development to improve quality of life.

Objectives

1. To ensure availability and accessibility of minimum mental health care for all in the foreseeable future, particularly to the most vulnerable and underprivileged sections of population
2. To encourage application of mental health knowledge in general health care and in social development
3. To promote community participation in the mental health services development and to stimulate efforts towards self-help in the community.

Strategies

1. Integration mental health with primary health care through the NMHP
2. Provision of tertiary care institutions for treatment of mental disorders
3. Eradicating stigmatization of mentally ill patients and protecting their rights through regulatory institutions like the Central Mental Health Authority, and State Mental Health Authority.

Mental Health Care

1. The mental morbidity requires priority in mental health treatment
2. Primary health care at village and subcenter level
3. At Primary Health Center level
4. At the District Hospital level
5. Mental Hospital and Teaching Psychiatric Units.

District Mental Health Program

Components

1. Training programs of all workers in the mental health team at the identified Nodal Institute in the state.

2. Public education in the mental health to increase awareness and reduce stigma.
3. For early detection and treatment, the OPD and indoor services are provided.
4. Providing valuable data and experience at the level of community to the state and center for future planning, improvement in service and research.

Agencies like World Bank and WHO have been contacted to support various components of the program. Funds are provided by the Government of India to the State Governments and the Nodal Institutes to meet the expenditure on staff, equipments, vehicles, medicine, stationary, contingencies, training, etc. for initial 5 years and thereafter they should manage themselves. Government of India has constituted Central Mental Health Authority to oversee the implementation of the Mental Health Act 1986. It provides for creation of State Mental Health Authority also to carry out the said functions.

The National Human Rights Commission also monitors the conditions in the mental hospitals along with the Government of India and the states are currently acting on the recommendation of the joint studies conducted to ensure quality in delivery of mental care.

Thrust areas for 10th Five Year Plan

1. District Mental Health program in an enlarged and more effective form covering the entire country.
2. Streamlining/modernization of mental hospitals in order to modify their present custodial role.
3. Upgrading department of psychiatry in medical colleges and enhancing the psychiatry content of the medical curriculum at the undergraduate as well as postgraduate level.
4. Strengthening the Central and State Mental Health Authorities with a permanent secretariat. Appointment of medical officers at state headquarters in order to make their monitoring role more effective;
5. Research and training in the field of community mental health, substance abuse and child/adolescent psychiatric clinics.

Comments

1. For the first time in the last 40 years mental health has been chosen as the theme for the World Health Day 2001: "Mental Health: Stop Exclusion-Date to Care", Why? The recent evidence for the importance of mental health has been so striking that the WHO decided to give it a priority during year 2001, the beginning of 21st century.
2. There is no initiative from the mental health professional to take active part in this program. Most of them are not aware of the program.
3. There is shortage of professional manpower and training programs are not able to meet the demand in providing all medical private practitioners and medical officers.

4. Appropriate mental health can be provided at the subcenter and village level by minimum training of the health workers that will help in providing comprehensive health care at the most peripheral level.
5. The targets set for the program are not achieved till today after lapse of more than one decade. This indicates that there is a poor commitment of the government, psychiatrists, and community at large.
6. The program has given more emphasis on the curative services to the mental disorders and preventive measures are largely ignored. More public awareness programs are required.
7. The medical care in the hospitals are custodial in nature and this needs to be changed to a therapeutic approach.

PSYCHIATRIC REHABILITATION

- A person is considered to have disabilities when he/she persistently cannot perform up to the standards expected by the society.
- Psychiatric patients have three kinds of disabilities:
    - Impairment of function directly due to psychiatric symptoms, e.g. persistent hallucinations, social withdrawal, slowness in behavior;
    - Social disadvantages, e.g. unemployment, homelessness, stigma attached to being a psychiatric patient;
    - Adverse psychological reactions, e.g. low self-esteem, helplessness, hopelessness.
- Psychiatric rehabilitation includes two processes:
    - Identifying, preventing, or minimizing the above three disabilities;
    - Helping the person to develop and use his/her assets.
- Rehabilitation also involves community nurses, social workers, occupational therapists, and even voluntary workers.

Facilities

Psychiatric rehabilitation facilities can be divided into non-residential and residential
- Non-residential facilities include psychiatric day hospitals, psychiatric day training centers, sheltered workshops, and social clubs
- Residential facilities include halfway houses, compassionate rehousing, and long stay care homes.

Inpatient care

- With provision for occupational and social services
- Sheltered work and recreational facilities in the walking distance.

Day Hospital

- Patients attend for assessment, supervision of treatment and social activities.

Outpatient Clinics

- In the community to avoid missing of appointments
- Follow up by a community nurse.

Psychiatric Day Hospital

- As implied by its name 'hospital', the primary aim of this facility is treatment of psychiatric illnesses rather than rehabilitation of patients' disabilities
- Hence, the key professionals involved are doctors and nurses
- The advantages of day treatment over inpatient treatment include more contact with the community, less risk of dependency, less social stigma, and less family disruption.

Psychiatric Day Training Center

- Aim of day training centers is rehabilitation of patients' disabilities, rather than the treatment of psychiatric illnesses
- Hence, there are no doctors and nurses
- The key professionals involved are social workers and occupational therapists.
- Patients are usually expected to stay in the center for rehabilitative training for about 9 months.
- While receiving training in the center, patients have to return to psychiatric outpatient clinics for follow-up from time to time.

Sheltered Workshop

- Aim of this facility is for patients to work, rather than to receive rehabilitation
- This is reflected by the fact that patients can earn salaries, though meagre, for their production in the workshop, whereas in all other rehabilitation facilities, patients have to pay fees instead
- Patients work in sheltered workshops instead of finding open employment because they cannot perform up to the standards of normal people
- Compared with psychiatric day training center, sheltered workshop has a much lower staff-to-patient ratio and no occupational therapist
- Patients' works are supervised mainly by non-trained staff
- Many psychiatric patients receive rehabilitative training in psychiatric day hospital or day training center first
- After they have acquired sufficient occupational skills, they are then referred to sheltered workshop to practise these skills.

Social Clubs

- Social club does not aim to rehabilitate patients actively
- It mainly provides recreational activities for patients to socialize among themselves, to prevent patients from idling alone
- The club may also organize educational groups for club members selectively.

Halfway House

- Halfway house is a residential rehabilitation facility
- It is indicated when patients have adverse home environment or no home at all, or when patients need rehabilitation in their social and domestic skills
- Halfway houses have no occupational therapist and do not aim to train patients' occupational skills
- Residents usually go out to work in the day time.

Compassionate Rehousing

- This facility is indicated for rehabilitated patients who cannot return to their families but who do not need to be placed in institutions
- Used by Government of Hong Kong.

Long-stay Care Home

- It is indicated for socially disabled mental patients who cannot live independently and who need care
- It is expected that only a small proportion of its residents can eventually be discharged back to the community
- Long-stay care homes differ from psychiatric hospitals
- Here, a few hours of may be made available per week.

Correctional Homes

- For young child who has been found guilty of an offence that would be categorized as a crime if committed by an adult
- Many are boys between the age of 15–17 years
- For example, Correctional home at Madiwala, Bengaluru.

Psychosocial Rehabilitation Institutions in India

- Center for Rehabilitation—CIP: Rehabilitation services in the form of Occupational Therapy Unit from 1922
- NIMHANS—Comprehensive care and rehabilitation for psychiatric and neuropatients, NIMHANS created a separate department in 1985
- The Richmond Fellowship Society (India)
- Vishwas Day Care Center with vocational training
- VIMHANS (Vidyasagar Institute of Mental Health and Neuro-Sciences), New Delhi.

Institutions in Kerala

- IMHANS is an autonomous institution established by the State Government of Kerala in 1983
- Mental Health Center, Kozhikode
- Mental Health Center, Thrissur and Thiruvananthapuram
- Shraddha Rehabilitation Foundation, Mumbai

- Institute of Psychiatry, Kilpauk, Chennai
- Kusumagiri Mental Health Center (KMHC).

INSTITUTIONALIZATION VS DE INSTITUTIONALIZATION

Institutionalization

Institutionalization refers to the process of committing an individual to a mental hospital.

In Europe and North America, the trend of putting the mentally ill into mental hospitals began as early as 17th century and hospitals often focused more on restraining or controlling inmates than on curing them.

Issues of institutionalization
- Overcrowding in institutions.
    - Failure of institutional treatment to cure most mental illness
    - Unable to adjust to independent living
    - Increasing popularity of deinstitutionalization
    - Increasing growth of community mental health services.

Deinstitutionalization

History

By the beginning of the 20th century, ever increasing admissions had resulted in serious overcrowding. Funding was often cut, especially during periods of economic decline, and during wartime in particular many patients starved to death. Asylums became notorious for poor living conditions, lack of hygiene, overcrowding and ill treatment and abuse of patients.

The first community based alternatives were suggested and tentatively implemented in the 1920s and 1930s, although asylum numbers continued to increase up to the 1950s. The movement of deinstitutionalization, came to the fore in various countries in the 1950s and 1960s.

Deinstitutionalization is the process of replacing long-stay psychiatric hospitals with less isolated community mental health service for those diagnosed with mental disorder.

Aim

- To reduce population size of mental institutions
- To remove institutional processes from mental hospitals that may create dependency, hopelessness and other maladaptive behaviors.

Chapter 16

Mental Disorders for Special People

MENTAL DISORDERS IN WOMEN

Some Facts about Women's Mental Health

- Recorded rates of anxiety and depression are one and a half to two times higher in women than in men.
- One study showed that 57% of those attending emergency departments for self-harm were women.
- About 13–15% of new mothers experience postnatal depression.
- Women in custody have a high level of psychological disturbance – 78%, compared with 15% in women in the general adult female population.
- Nearly two-thirds of women on remand have a diagnosis of depression. More than 40% have attempted suicide before entering prison. More than twice as many have an eating disorder compared with women in the general population.
- One in four women will experience intimate partner (domestic) violence (IPV) in their lifetime. Depression affects nearly half of women exposed to IPV, and post-traumatic stress disorder (PTSD) affects almost two-thirds.
- About 90% of the 1.6 million people in the UK who have an eating disorder are female.

Gender Inequality and Risks to Women's Mental Health

Gender inequality in society leads to differences in the life experiences of men and women, which affect mental health in different ways. Gender inequality is described as a system that tends to give more advantages to men in terms of employment, status and ownership. Women are much more often expected to look after others in the home or in society, often doing work that is undervalued and unpaid or poorly paid.

Some risk factors for mental health problems affect women more often than men. These include gender-based violence, social and economic disadvantage, low income and income inequality, low or subordinate social status and rank, and major responsibility for the care of others.

Gender Differences in Mental Health Disorders

Women receive more services than men for mental health problems at the level of primary care, though this difference is less at the level of secondary care (specialist and hospital treatment). It is difficult to know whether more mental

health problems are diagnosed in women at primary care level because they seek help more often than men, or because they actually experience more distress.

According to another WHO report, there is little difference in the prevalence of mental health disorders between men and women, but the types of disorders and the stages of life at which mental health problems are most likely to be diagnosed differ. In childhood, boys are more often identified as having mental disorders, such as attention-deficit hyperactivity disorder, and substance abuse is more common. Young women experience more depression, self-harm and eating disorders. In adulthood, women are far more likely to be diagnosed with depression. Psychotic disorders such as schizophrenia and bipolar disorder are similarly likely in both sexes. In old age, women are more likely to be diagnosed with depression and psychoses.

Women are more likely than men to have more than one disorder, which increases disability.

Diagnoses Most Commonly given to Women

Depression

First episodes of depression are more frequent in women than men, and are likely to result from a mixture of social, psychological and biological factors. Fluctuating hormone levels may partly explain the higher rates of depression in women; however, hormones are likely to affect other aspects of women's lives, such as their general health, relationships and living environment, and with social factors, such as the position of women in society and the value placed on women's roles, rather than being the sole cause of depression.

First episodes of depression in women have been linked to the onset of puberty and menstruation, childbirth, and the transition to menopause. Depression is more frequent in married than never-married women, and in unsupported mothers.

Anxiety

Anxiety is more frequent in women than in men, though this may partially reflect the relative unwillingness of men to seek help. Men are more likely to turn to drugs or alcohol (in particular) to cope with stress problems, and are more likely to develop substance abuse problems than women.

Anxiety problems, including panic, agoraphobia, obsessive–compulsive disorder (OCD) and PTSD, are reported up to twice as often by women as by men. People with PTSD may have a range of symptoms, including re-experiencing painful events, avoidance, muscular and emotional tension, depression, emotional numbing, drug or alcohol misuse and anger.

Eating Disorders

Disordered eating patterns, such as compulsive dieting or eating, with or without induced vomiting and purging, can affect men and women, but the overwhelming

majority of those affected are girls and women aged between 14 and 25 years. Girls are becoming weight conscious as young as five years of age. Since, eating disorders are more common in developed and industrialized countries, it seems likely that the main causes are social and psychological, and relate to cultural pressures on young women to look slim. Young women from other ethnicities and cultures living in the UK and USA also acquire eating disorders, and may be at greater risk than white women.

Self-harm and Suicidal Behavior

The majority of people who self-harm are young women. Self-harming behavior is also significant among minority groups discriminated against by society. Someone who has mental health problems is more likely to self-harm. So those who are dependent on drugs or alcohol, or who are faced with a number of major life problems. Women are most likely to self-harm by cutting or poisoning themselves.

The majority of people who self-harm are not suicidal, but, people who self-harm are at higher risk of suicide than any other group. Men have a higher rate of suicide than women—17.4 men per 100,000 compared to 5.3 women. Reasons for this include the idea that women form more socially supportive networks than men, since isolation appears to be a factor in suicide. However, deaths by hanging have increased among young women in recent years.

Borderline Personality Disorder (BPD)

The majority (70%) of people diagnosed with BPD are women, and suicide rates are high among this group (10%). BPD has been linked to a history of trauma in childhood and PTSD.

Diagnoses Related to Reproductive Functions

Hormonal and reproductive changes can contribute to some mental health problems, and some diagnoses that women receive relate to aspects of their reproductive functions, including menstruation, pregnancy and childbirth, and menopause.

Premenstrual Syndrome

Premenstrual hormonal changes have been linked to problems that can range from mild feelings of depression or irritation to, very rarely, premenstrual dysphoric disorder, characterized by anxiety, depression, insomnia, food cravings and feelings of being out of control.

Perinatal Mental Disorders

Women are particularly vulnerable to mental health problems in the time just before and after childbirth—the perinatal period. The main types of mental health problem that arise are:

- Depression in pregnancy
- Postnatal blues
- Postnatal depression
- Puerperal psychosis.

While pregnancy is widely believed to reduce depression, some studies have found that depression in pregnancy is more widespread than expected, especially in the third trimester.

'Postnatal blues' is a normal emotional change that occurs in up to 50% of women after childbirth, and is thought to be linked to rapid changes in hormones. It is usually brief, although it is advised that women are monitored to ensure that this is not the start of postnatal depression.

Postnatal depression and puerperal psychosis are no different from depression or psychosis experienced at any other time. Some experts believe that giving birth acts as a major stress factor that can trigger the onset of these disorders in women who are predisposed to them. Postnatal depression can begin in the weeks following childbirth, or up to a year afterwards. The woman may feel low in mood and energy, worried about her child, and unable to sleep, or even have thoughts about abandoning or harming her child.

While 13–15% of women experience postnatal depression, puerperal psychosis is much rarer, affecting only about 1 in 1000. It is a serious mental illness that can develop in a woman who has recently given birth, usually with no obvious cause. The baby may be healthy and wanted, and the birth is not unusually complicated.

For women who already have mental disorders, such as schizophrenia or bipolar disorder, pregnancy can bring additional stress. Some women with bipolar disorder may experience a worsening of their symptoms during pregnancy and after the birth.

Diagnoses Women Receive Less Frequently

Schizophrenia and Bipolar Disorder

While there are no marked differences in the incidence of schizophrenia between the sexes, women tend to be older than men by three to six years when first diagnosed, often in their late 20s, and there is a further peak of onset in women after 45 years of age. There are also differences in the types of symptoms women experience and in rates of recovery. Researchers therefore recommend a gender-sensitive approach to the diagnosis and management of schizophrenia.

The type of bipolar disorder experienced by women is usually characterized by mild 'hypomanic' episodes, but with a greater burden of depression; researchers also recommend a gender-sensitive approach.

Substance Dependence

Substance (drug and alcohol) dependence is more common in men but the experience of substance dependence is often different for women. Traditionally,

a greater social stigma is attached to women who are dependent on illegal drugs or alcohol, which can lead them to hide their problems, and choose not to access health or social care services. Women who are lone parents are particularly likely to hide their problems through fear that they may lose custody of their children. In these situations, substance dependence and coexisting mental health problems are likely to become more severe over time, with serious consequences for a woman's health and wellbeing.

Women are more likely than men to become dependent on prescription medication, including antidepressants and tranquillisers (for anxiety or use as sleeping pills). This is partly because women are more frequently diagnosed with anxiety and depression and given medication to treat these conditions.

Social Factors that affect Women's Mental Health

Far more women than men use primary care services for mental health problems, and one reason suggested is that women are more likely to report symptoms of common mental health problems. Rates of undiagnosed depression could be equally high in men, but evidence suggests that men are less likely to talk about their problems or consult a doctor about their mental health. By contrast, women are more likely to acknowledge their mental distress and to seek help.

Economic Issues

Some mental disorders, such as depression, are more common among those living in poverty. Women are more likely to be poor because their jobs are likely to be lower paid, they are more likely to work part-time, to take time out of the labor market to bring up children, to be lone parents, and, because of their different working history, likely to receive a lower pension. This goes a longway to explain why rates of depression are higher in women.

Trauma, Violence and Abuse in Childhood or Adulthood

Gender-based violence is strongly linked with mental health issues, including depression, anxiety and stress-related syndromes, substance misuse and suicide.

Up to 13% of children experience sexual abuse, physical abuse, neglect, or disruption such as being in care, with slightly higher figures for girls than boys. One in four adult women experience IPV (domestic violence). IPV is defined as any incident of threatening behavior, violence or abuse (psychological, physical, sexual, financial or emotional) between adults who are (or who have been) intimate partners or family members, regardless of gender or sexuality. This includes so-called 'honor killings' that are of concern in black and minority ethnic (BME) communities.

Women are much more likely than men to experience repeated and severe forms of IPV, although this is not always evident in statistical summaries such as home office studies, which may focus on single incidents rather than on repeated abuse. Women are also more likely to experience sexual abuse and violence, and their experience is more likely to have a long-lasting psychological/

emotional impact or result in injury or death. In some cases, mental illness, such as schizophrenia, can increase the risk of IPV.

Experience of IPV can lead to feelings of guilt and shame, anxiety, depression, low self-esteem, lack of confidence, vulnerability to abusive relationships, inability to trust people, anger, sexual difficulties and self-hate. Women can also experience physical symptoms related to abuse, such as abdominal pain, insomnia and headaches. Further, these problems can lead to the diagnosis of a wide range of mental disorders, including PTSD, BPD, self-harm, suicide (or suicide attempts), multiple personality disorder, mania, bulimia, eating disorders and substance abuse.

Family and Social Roles

For some women, family life may contribute to mental distress. Many women have primary or sole care of children, and women are more likely than men to take on caring responsibilities (e.g. for older family members). Women also tend to work in part-time jobs, and are over-represented in low paid occupations and sectors such as teaching and care work. The low social status traditionally associated with domestic and caring work can damage feelings of self-worth, while the stresses of overwork, extensive responsibilities and feeling undervalued can damage women's mental health. While the extent of gender-based disadvantages varies according to social class and ethnicity, it has been argued that women bear the brunt of reconciling paid work with family life.

Women who are mothers, or who want to have children, can experience particular barriers to the use of mental health services. They may avoid disclosing their problems for fear of losing custody of their children, leave hospital sooner than they otherwise would, in order to look after children, or find themselves unable to use services because of childcare commitments.

Younger Women

Childhood and adolescent mental health difficulties are strongly correlated with mental health problems in adulthood. Problems that are more likely to be diagnosed in women than men, such as eating disorders, BPD and self-harm, often start in teenage years or early adulthood.

Teenage girls and young women are at high risk for traumatic experiences such as sexual abuse, rape and domestic violence. As discussed above (Trauma, violence and abuse in childhood or adulthood), girls who experience sexual or physical abuse are more likely to develop mental health problems later in life.

Older Women

Issues around old age are particularly relevant to women's mental health.
- Because of their longer life expectancy, women make up the larger part of this demographic group. Among all older people, women are more likely than men to be diagnosed with a mental health problem.

- Higher rates of mental ill-health have been associated with the greater social and personal pressures that women often face in later life—isolation and poverty are more common in older women than in older men.
- Older women are less likely to have a company or personal pension, and are more likely to be reliant on state pensions.
- Older women are less likely to be drivers or to have access to a car.
- Bereavement, chronic physical illness and institutional care are also likely to impact upon older women's mental health.

However, the higher rates of diagnosed mental health problems in older women may partly reflect the fact that women are, in general, more likely than men to acknowledge their distress and seek appropriate help.

Women in Prison and Secure Psychiatric Services

Women in prison often have complex problems. A high proportion have had adverse childhood experiences, problems at school and poor employment records. Rates of mental disorder and substance abuse are high, and being in prison can increase women's problems, as they may be separated from their children and social networks, and they may be victimized. Women in prison experience higher rates of mental disorder than women in the community or men in prison, and rates are higher still for remand prisoners. Rates of self-harm and suicide are high among women in prison.

Women in secure psychiatric hospitals are in a minority, but women are proportionately more likely than men to be sent to such hospitals for criminal behavior, or transferred from another hospital because of a behavioral disorder. They have had similar adverse experiences growing up to women in prison generally, though fewer are mothers. Self-harm and substance abuse are common among this group.

Women Refugees and Asylum Seekers

Being a refugee or asylum seeker can be traumatic for both men and women, but particular experiences such as rape are more common among women. Women who are refugees or asylum seekers may arrive from traumatic situations to find themselves detained, which has been described as 'retraumatization'. They are physically examined, but are rarely asked if they are victims of torture; even if they are asked and the response is 'yes', often nothing is done.

Women in detention centers are almost inevitably depressed, having fled from their home countries, and having often been persecuted, tortured or raped, and are in fear of being deported back to the countries they have fled.

Race, Ethnicity and Mental Health

Women from BME groups in the UK may experience the dual impact of gender inequality within their family or community setting, and alienation from mental health services. The high levels of suicide and self-harm among young South Asian women are indications of this.

Specific groups of BME women are heavily represented in psychiatric diagnoses and service use; Pakistani and Bangladeshi women have higher rates of depression than both their male counterparts and White British women. Higher rates of psychosis (including bipolar disorder and schizophrenia) are diagnosed among Black Caribbean women than among women from other groups. It is argued that this may be partly because racism within society is reflected by racial stereotyping within mental health services. Many mental health service users from BME groups are also living in poverty, which is an important social factor in mental distress.

Sexuality

Lesbian and bisexual women tend to have higher rates of suicide, attempted suicide and suicidal thoughts, depression, anxiety and substance use disorders than heterosexual women. Such mental health issue may of course be unconnected with their sexuality, but there is evidence that social hostility, stigma and discrimination are contributing factors.

Social Factors that Support Women's Mental Health

Women are encouraged to become competent at relationships, and as a result are better than men at seeking help and dealing with the causes of their distress. They also tend to be better able to give and receive help from each other. Women who have strong family support, autonomy, and access to material resources that allow choice are better protected against developing mental health problems.

Physical and Mental Health Interactions

Physical and mental ill-health are linked in both men and women. People with chronic physical illnesses are at greater risk of developing mental health problems, particularly depression, while those with mental health problems are also more likely to have physical illnesses, such as heart or respiratory problems.

Medically Unexplained Symptoms

A range of physical problems are considered by doctors to be the physical manifestation of mental health problems, otherwise known as 'conversion symptoms' or 'somatization'. These include irritable bowel syndrome, fibromyalgia, and chronic pelvic pain. Studies show that medically unexplained symptoms such as these are two to three times more likely in women than in men. Research shows that a high proportion of people with such problems have experienced trauma, abuse or violence.

Unrecognized Physical Ill-health

An equally serious problem for women in mental distress is the lack of recognition for physical illnesses, because symptoms of physical illness may be wrongly seen as 'imagined' or psychosomatic. Research suggests that women with mental

health problems are more likely than other groups to have physical complaints disregarded, and requests for services denied. Studies have found that women with mental health problems have significantly more undetected medical problems than men, and that women with bipolar disorder (manic depression) are three times more likely than men to have undiagnosed medical problems.

Treatment and Services

Department of Health guidance on mainstreaming women's mental health has pointed out that women ultimately want services to adopt a 'whole person' approach to their care, treatment and rehabilitation, to value their strengths and abilities, and to recognize their potential for recovery, in the context of holistic assessment and care planning. Many areas of women's mental health are now also covered by guidance from the National Institute for Health and Clinical Excellence (NICE).

Anxiety and Depression

Too often, a diagnosis of anxiety or depression leads to medication as the first or only treatment option. Women with these issues have repeatedly asked for better access to talking therapies, and for opportunities to learn new skills and coping strategies. These preferences are reflected in current NICE guidelines for the treatment of both anxiety and depression, which state that talking therapies are the most likely treatment to produce lasting benefits, especially when combined with other forms of social support and self-help. Government investment in the improving access to psychological therapies program has increased the availability of short-term therapies such as cognitive behavior therapy (CBT) via primary care. Pilot programs show that over 60% of those accessing this CBT are women, and that the intervention shows some positive results in reducing levels of depression and anxiety.

Eating Disorders

Talking treatments, including family therapy and CBT, are widely advised for women with eating disorders. NICE guidance on treatment for anorexia advises structured and symptom-focused inpatient admission as a last resort, with psychological treatment rather than behavior modification. However, a lack of specialist eating disorder services across large areas of England and Wales means that local services often fall short of national standards.

Self-harm

For women who self-harm, NICE recommends full assessment of physical, psychological and social needs, by a professional with suitable training and in an atmosphere of respect and understanding. Treatment choices should include counseling and therapy. Women who have self-harmed severely should be referred to psychiatric services for further assessment, treatment and support, or taken into hospital in an emergency.

Borderline Personality Disorder

For women diagnosed with BPD, NICE recommends that a clearly structured, comprehensive multi-disciplinary care plan that includes short- and long-term goals is agreed with the client. The care plan should include psychological treatments of at least three months' duration, and plans to manage crises. No medications are specifically recommended for BPD. NICE and other agencies recommend a range of treatment options, including structured talking treatments, and medication for specific symptoms, such as transient psychotic episodes.

Perinatal Disorders

Women clearly benefit from support before and after childbirth. One study shows that counseling for women who are depressed when pregnant may help to prevent problems for the family after the baby is born. Other studies show that health visitors can provide valued listening and support to new mothers, and that individual, group and family support and counseling can help mothers to cope with postnatal depression and parenting problems.

NICE has produced guidance on perinatal (ante- and postnatal) mental health, which recommends that health professionals look out for those most at risk of developing a mental disorder, and ask questions to detect problems, such as depression, as early as possible. This ensures that psychological treatment can begin as early as possible if needed, within one month of initial assessment, and no longer than three months afterwards.

NICE guidance recommends that clinical networks are developed in each region to ensure that services for mothers and infants are better coordinated, and that help is available quickly when needed.

Treatment for Women Diagnosed with severe Mental Illnesses such as schizophrenia

Experts have argued that gender-aware treatment for women with diagnoses such as schizophrenia should mean doctors taking more account of women's practical and emotional needs and their social roles as partners, mothers, and professionals or employees. Women may need therapy and support focused on maintaining or re-establishing their roles, and perhaps will do better if they can receive help that does not separate them from their children, but helps them to cope better with parenting.

Women Who have Experienced Abuse or Violence

Guidance has been developed to help health professionals work with women who may be experiencing mental disorders as a result of abuse, violence or trauma. The first step is to ask questions to find out about these experiences. Some studies show that, despite guidance, many staff do not do this well, perhaps because of a lack of training and experience.

The World Psychiatric Association recommends that women who have been sexually abused and those who have strong preferences for female healthcare staff should be accommodated whenever possible, and emphasises that the evaluation of mental health problems in women must consider the full context of their lives, as distress often has social origins.

Diagnoses should not be stigmatizing, and the role of violence and discrimination in the genesis of mental health problems in women requires special consideration.

General Issues Relating to Medication

Side Effects and Interactions

Side effects of psychiatric medication that women in particular may find distressing include weight gain and hair loss. In addition, medications can interact with each other in problematic ways, for instance, some medications interact with the oral contraceptive pill.

Motherhood and Medication

While medication for antenatal and postnatal depression is an option, NICE guidance says that the risks of anti-depressant medication to the unborn child, or the infant through breast milk, should be explained, and talking treatments and self-help options should be explored.

The issue of medication is particularly important for women with schizophrenia or bipolar disorder who are mothers or who want to become mothers. Healthcare professionals need to work sensitively with women who are already on medication about whether or not it is safe and advisable to take a break from medication, taking into account the additional stresses of pregnancy and parenting, and the amount of support available. If this is considered possible, then experts advise tapering off the dose of medication in order to avoid the risk of damage to the developing fetus.

Safety Issues for Women in Psychiatric Hospitals

Sexual safety includes freedom from sexual harassment, exploitation, aggression and violence. Women are entitled to feel safe from physical harm or sexual harassment when in a mental health unit; there can be particular issues for women who have experienced sexual abuse or rape.

Separate sleeping, toilets and bathing accommodation for women in mental health units has been policy since 2000, and, according to the National Patient Safety Agency (NPSA), mental health units should be reconfigured to provide either a self-contained, women-only ward or solely single sex wards. Many, though not all, have done this. However, physical and sexual safety for women in mental health units is an ongoing issue, and the NPSA recommends better use of existing guidance and more training for staff to recognize and report incidents

such as sexual harassment, taking into account the physical and psychological harm caused.

Improving Mental Health Policy and Practice for Women

Since the Department of Health's report on women's mental health, policies to improve treatment of women have become part of mainstream work. A number of NHS trusts have developed mental health strategies for women, and, in the light of gender equality duty, many are now further updating and reviewing their policies.

Current priority areas for improvement according to a recent national report are:
- Health and wellbeing
- Supporting women in their roles as mothers, carers, employees and students
- Safety and freedom from threat of abuse or violence
- Justice and fairness for women who come into contact with the criminal justice system
- Women's participation, particularly empowering women from BME communities.

Many of the initiatives to improve services for women, however, still have a long-way to go. Women have been calling for more support for self-help and alternatives to medicalized treatments for many years, but in most cases these alternatives are not well supported financially, and are usually left to the voluntary sector to provide, and therefore not universally available.

MENTAL DISORDERS IN ELDERS

Aging is not merely the passage of time. It is the manifestation of biological events that occur over a span of time. It is important to recognize that people age differently. The aging body does change. Some systems slow down, while others lose their "fine tuning." As a general rule, slight, gradual changes are common, and most of these are not problems to the person who experiences them. Sudden and dramatic changes might indicate serious health problems.

Biological Aspect of Aging

Individuals are unique in their psychological and physical aging process. As the individual ages, there is a quantitative loss of cells and changes in many of enzymatic activities within cells resulting in a diminished responsiveness to biological demands made on the body. Age related a change occurs at different rate in different people.

Nervous System

- The brain atrophies as a result of aging process. The brain weight decreases, decrease in enzymes, protein and lipids in brain tissue.

- There is shrinkage of large neurons resulting in loss of large neurons with an increase in smaller neurons.
- There is alterations in the amount for some neurotransmitters.
- Clinical changes due to the above are decreased sensation of vibrations (particularly in legs), less brisk deep tendon reflexes with ankle reflex absent entirely and a decreased ability for upward gaze.
- Functional changes include slowing of response to tasks and the increase in time to recover from physical exertion.
- Cognitive changes include memory loss, decrease in perceptual ability and decrease in proficiency.

Sensory Changes

1. Eyes

- The eye's external changes give evidence of advancing age. These changes result from loss of orbital fat, loss of elastic tissue and decreased muscle tone.
- The skin around the eyes darkens and wrinkles referred to as "crow's feet" appear.
- Xanthomas (cutaneous deposits of lipid material) found at the inner portion of the lid; these may indicate elevated blood lipid levels.
- The cornea flattens which reduces the refractory power.
- The retina of older individual becomes thinner because of fewer neural cells and receives only 1/3rd of the amount of light that of a younger person. Due to this problem in reading, not able to see in dim light and also have difficulty in color perception.
- The lens of the eye loses its elasticity and increases in density.

2. Ear

- Cerumen gland are reduced in number dry and hard ear wax, along with itching.
- Degenerative changes occur in ossicles contributing to hearing loss
- Loss of cochlear hair cells leading to hearing loss; Inner ear changes affect the auditory processing system leading to auditory processing disorder and a peripheral hearing sensitivity loss.
- Presbycusis is the term used to describe hearing loss associated with normal aging.

3. Taste and Smell

- Very rarely the capacity to smell diminishes;
- Taste perception and taste discrimination decreases as the age advances.

Integumentary System

- Systemic decrease in circulation, loss of cells and loss of elastic collagen fibers and muscle mass.

- The number of pressure and light touch sensors decreases with age
- Subcutaneous fat atrophies on the face, hands, shins and soles; whereas it hypertrophies on the abdomen (in men) and thighs (in women)
- Immune, vascular and thermoregulatory responses of the skin decrease with age
- Loss of hair color and thinning of pubic, axillary and scalp hair.

Cardiovascular System

- Collagen and lipid deposits increase intercellularity in the heart muscle.
- Lipofuscin, a yellow-brown granular material accumulates in the myocardial cell.
- Valves of the heart becomes thicker and more rigid as a result of calcification.
- The SA node is infiltrated by fat and connective tissue resulting in a decrease in the heart's ability to regulate the rate of SA node, also causing a slowing of electrical impulses through the AV tissue.
- There is 10% decrease in the number of pacemaker cells in the SA node by age 75 years. Many of the arrhythmias seen in the older person are a result of either the decrease in pacemaker cells or the infiltration of fat in the SA node.

Respiratory System

- Degeneration of the intervertebral discs leading to development of kyphosis and scoliosis
- The trachea and large bronchi are also increased in diameter because of the calcified cartilage changes
- The muscles involved in respiration weaken with age. It results in less forceful contraction which decreases inspiratory and expiratory effort.
- The combination of increased stiffness of the chest wall and decreased muscle strength results in less efficient breathing.
- Older people depend more on accessory abdominal muscles to compensate for weakened thoracic muscles.

Musculoskeletal System

- Bone resorption takes place without the successful formation of new bone mass leading to gradual bone loss.
- Loss of trabecular bone leads to compression fractures in vertebral column.
- Reduction in cortical thickness and increased porosity results in progressive cortical thinning.
- In aging, the increased parathyroid hormone, decreased vitamin D and calcitonin also play role in calcium loss in older people.
- In women, estrogen deficiency, calcium malabsorption, lifestyle factors (calcium intake and exercise) can result in bone loss. Aging brings decline in numbers of muscles resulting in reduced muscle mass.
- The muscle strength also reduces especially due to lack of exercise.

Urinary System

- In men, BPH is associated with aging leads to urinary incontinence (dribbling).
- In women, estrogen deficiency causes changes in the squamous epithelium of the distal urethral and vaginal wall, a decrease in the vaginal muscular tone and vascular profusion. These changes contribute to urinary incontinence.
- Increasing age is also associated with an increase in involuntary bladder contractions, a reduction in bladder capacity and an increase in residual volume. These contribute to development of incontinence in older adults.
- Weak pelvic muscles causes stress incontinence.

Gastrointestinal System

- Teeth become brittle; there is resorption of bone in the jaw leading to loosening of teeth, increased infections of teeth and gums and eventual loss of teeth.
- Difficult to chew food because of loose teeth.
- Common bile duct undergo progressive dilatation with age.
- Presence of gall stones increases with age.
- Liver weight and size decreases with age
- There is decrease in number of hepatic cells and as a result, a diminished capacity for metabolism of drugs and hormones.

Reproductive System

Changes in Women

- Menopause begins between the ages of 45 to 50 years. The cessation of ovarian secretion of estrogen and progesterone is the major physiologic event of menopause. Women may experience hot flashes due to vasomotor instability. Also another associated feature of menopause is bone loss leading to osteoporosis.
- Decrease in estrogen production leads to reduced vaginal lubrication, the vaginal mucosa becomes thin and the vagina shortens in length and width. Due to this reason, the sexual arousal is reduced which results in painful intercourse and vulvo-vaginitis.

Changes in Men

Erectile ability undergoes changes. Takes longer time for erection, amount of semen is reduced and the intensity of ejaculation is lessened.
It is not clear that whether the increase in impotence is age related.

Psychological Aspects of Aging

Memory Functioning

- Short-term memory deteriorate with age, long-term memory does not show similar changes.

- A well educated and mentally active person does not exhibit such changes in faster rate.
- The time required for memory scanning is longer for both recent and remote recall among older people.
- This can be attributed to social or health factors (stress, fatigue, illness), but it can also occur with certain physiological changes due to aging (decreased blood flow to the brain).

Intellectual Functioning

- Fluid abilities or abilities involved in solving novel problems, tend to decline from adult period to old age.
- High degree of regularity in intellectual function present on most of the old age people
- Intellectual abilities of older people do not decline, but do become obsolete.
- Their formal educational experience is reflected in their intelligence performance.

Learning Ability

- The ability to learn is not decline by age.
- The slowing of reaction time with age and over arousal of central nervous system are noted in old age. It may lead to lower level of performance in tasks which requires high efficiency.
- Ability to learn continue throughout the life, although strongly influenced by personal interests and preferences.
- Accuracy of performances diminishes.

Adaptation to the Tasks of Ageing

1. Loss and grief
   - By the time individuals reach 60–70 years of age, they have experienced numerous losses, and mourning has become a life long process.
   - It is impossible for some of the older age people to complete the grief process in response to one loss before the other loss occurs.
   - Because the grief is cumulative, this can result in bereavement over load.
   - This can further predispose to depression.
2. Attachment to others
   - The need for attachment is consistent through out the life span
   - Well being of senior citizens can be contributed through socialization and companionship.
3. Maintenance of self-identity
   - Self-concept and self-identity appears to remain stable over life-time.
   - Factors which contribute to good psychosocial adjustment are sustained family relationships, maturity of the ego defenses, absence of depressive disorder and absence of alcoholism.

4. Dealing with death
   - Death anxiety among the elderly is more of a myth than reality
   - The feeling of abandment, pain and loss may leads to fear or anxiety in elderly.
5. Psychiatric disorders
   - The later life constitute a time of especially high risk for emotional distress
   - Dementia, depressive disorders, delirium, sleep disorders, etc. are the most common psychiatric illness seen among elderly.

Sociocultural Aspects of Aging

- Old age brings many important socially induced changes, some of those changes have the potential for negative effect on both the physical and mental well-being of older persons.
- They want protection from hazards and weariness of everyday tasks
- They want to treated with respect and dignity and also want to die with respect and dignity.
- In developing countries and Asian countries' the aged are awarded a position of honor, that place emphasize on family cohesiveness.
- In industrialized countries many negative stereotyped perspectives on aging still persisting, aged are always tires or sick, slow and forgetful, isolated and lonely, unproductive, etc.
- Emplacement is one of the area where the aged faces discrimination. Although compulsory retirements has been eliminated, discrimination still persist in hiring and promoting the aged employees.
- The status of elderly may improve with time as the number of elder person increases worldwide.

Sexual Aspects of Ageing

Physical Changes

a. Changes in female
- Menopause may begin anytime during the 40s or early 50s
- Gradual decline in the functioning of the ovaries and subsequent reduction in the production of estrogen.
- The walls of the vagina become thin and inelastic and vaginal lubrication decreases.
- Orgasmic uterine contractions become spastic.
- All these changes result in vaginal burning, pelvic aching, irritability, etc
- In some women these changes result in avoidance of sexual intercourse
- These symptoms are more likely to occur with infrequent intercourse of only one time a month or less.
- Regular and more frequent sexual activity result in a greater capacity for sexual performance.

b. Changes in male
- Testosterone production decline gradually as the age increases
- As a result of these hormonal changes the erection takes place slowly and requires more genital stimulation to achieve.
- The volume of ejaculate decreases and the force of ejaculation lessens
- The testis become smaller, but most men continue to produce viable sperm well into old age.

Sexual Behavior in Elderly
- Sexual activity can continue and well preserve till the age of late 70s and 80s for both males and females who have regular opportunities for sexual expression
- As the sexual practices continues frequently, the sexual capacity can prolong
- Studies reveal that for healthy men and women with healthy partners, sexual activity will probably continue throughout life if they had a positive attitude about sex when they were young.

Chapter 17

Crisis Situation

STRESS AND COPING

Definition

Stress is defined as any factor that brings about a response or changes within a person.

Stress is how the body reacts to a stressor, real or imagined, a stimulus that causes stress.

Stressor is the stimuli proceeding or precipitating a change.

Stress may be linked to external factors such as:
- The state of the world, the country or any community to which you belong
- Unpredictable events
- The environment in which you live or work
- Work itself
- Family.

Stress can also come from your own:
- Irresponsible behavior
- Poor health habit
- Negative attitudes and feelings
- Unrealistic expectations
- Perfectionism.

Kinds of Stressors

External stressors:
- Physical environment
- Social interaction with people
- Life events which you have no control over (death in the family).

Internal stressors:
- Personal lifestyle choice
- Personality traits
- Individual thought process (negativity, over analyzing, etc).

External physical stressors include unpleasant environmental conditions such as pain, hot cold temperature infections or inflammation.

External psychological stressors are such things as poor working conditions or abusive relationships.

Internal psychological stressors include intense worry about money, a relationship problem or your self-image. Internal psychological stress can often

Model of Stress

General Adaptation Synorome Model

Selye labeled universal response to stressors the general adaptation syndrome (GAS).
Physiological response occurs in three stages (Fig. 7.1).

  i. Alarm reaction
     Alarm is the first stage. When the threat or stressor is identified or realized, the body's stress response is a state of alarm. During this stage, adrenaline will be produced in order to bring about the fight or flight response.
  ii. Stage of resistance
     Resistance is the second stage. If the stressor persists, it become necessary to attempt some means of coping with the stress. Although the body begins to try to adapt to the strains or demands of the environment, the body cannot keep this up indefinitely, so its resources are gradually depleted.
  iii. Stage of exhaustion
     Exhaustion is the third and final stage in the GAS model. At this point, all of the body's resources are eventually depleted and the body is unable to maintain normal function. At this point the initial autonomic nervous system symptoms may reappear. If stage three is extended, long-term damage may result as the capacity of gland, especially the adrenal gland, and the immune system is exhausted and function is impaired resulting in decompensation.

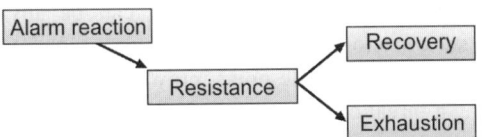

Figure 17.1: The general adaptation syndrome

Lazarus's Cognitive Appraisal Model

Lazarus argued that in order for a psychosocial situation to be stressful, it must be apprised as such. He argued that cognitive processes of appraisal are central in determining whether a situation is potentially threatening, constitutes a harm/loss, a challenge or is benign.

The primary appraisal is influenced by both person and environmental factors and triggers the selection of coping processes. Problem focused coping is directed at managing the problem, while emotion focused coping processes are directed at managing the negative emotions. Secondary appraisal refers to the evaluation of the resources available to cope with the problem and may alter the primary appraisal.

1. Hypothalamus
2. Posterior pituitary
   ↑ ADH →↑ H_2O
   Reabsorption ↓ urine
   Output
3. Anterior pituitary
   ↑ ACTH → Adrenal cortex
   ↑ Protein catabolism
   ↑ Fat catabolism
   ↑ Aldosterone ↑→Na reabsorption
   → H_2O reabsorption
   ↓ Urine all put
   ↑ Potassium excretion
4. Sympathetic nervous system and adrenal medulla
   ↑ Epinephrine → ↑ HR
   ↑ O_2 intake
   ↑ Blood glucose
   ↑ Mental acuity
   ↑ Norepinephrine→ ↑ Blood how to skeletal muscle
   ↑ Arterial blood pressure
5. Fight or flight response

1. Stabilization
2. Hormonal levels return to normal
3. Parasympathetic nervous system activity
4. Adaptation to stressors

1. ↑ Physiological response as noted in the alarm
2. ↓ Energy level
3. ↓ Physiological adaptation
4. Death

Stresses can also be defined as short-term (acute) or long-term (chronic)

Acute stress: Acute stress is the reaction to an immediate threat commonly known as fight or flight response. The threat can be any situation that is experienced, even subconsciously or falsely as a danger.

Common acute stressors include noise, crowding, isolation, hunger, danger, infection, imagining a threat or remembering a dangerous events.

Chronic stress: In day-to-day life a person faces different stressful situations, which are not short lived. The stress becomes chronic when an individual tries to suppress it.

Common chronic stressors include:

- Ongoing highly pressured work
- Long-term relationship problems
- Loneliness
- Persistent financial worries.

Kinds of Stress

Positive stress: A positive reaction towards an events. It is termed as 'ustress'. It has a positive effect spurring motivation and awareness, providing the stimulation to cope with challenging situations. It also provides the sense of urgency and alertness needed for survival when confronting threading situations

Negative stress: A negative reaction towards a particular event. It is termed as distress. It is a contributory factor in minor condition such as headaches, digestive problems, skin complaints, insomnia and ulcers.

Coping Strategy

Coping strategies refer to the specific efforts, both behavioral and psychological that people employ to minimize stressful events.

Strategies of Coping with Stress

- Get organized: Coping with stress is all about planning. You can plan to fail or plan to succeed. Organize time/or work, family, hobbies, spiritual time, time with friends and time alone, time for exercise and time for relaxation.
- Visualize the best outcome: Coping with stress is knowing how to deal with a stressful situation before it occurs. Rehearse how you are going to handle it. Picture yourself being successful in coping with stress.
- Do not postpone actions: One of the best strategies for coping with stress is not to put off actions until tomorrow if you can do it today. Coping with stress becomes more difficult when you defer. Do your least favorite chores first, followed by rewards.
- Be realistic: Set realistic goals. Emphasize quality over quantity. Work at a leisurely pace, taking breaks often.
- Sleep, eat an exercise: Coping with stress is all about treating your body properly. Eat food that nourish you, exercise and get plenty of sleep.

Unhealthy Ways of Coping with Stress

These coping strategies may temporarily reduce stress, but they cause more damage in the long run.
- Smoking
- Drinking too much
- Over eating or under eating
- Using pills or drugs to relax
- Sleeping too much
- Withdrawing from friends, family and activities
- Zoning out for hours in front of the TV or computer
- Taking out your stress on others (lashing out, angry outbursts, physical violence).

Dealing with Stressful Situation (4 A's)

Change the situation
- Avoid the stressor
- Alter the stressor

Change the reaction
- Adapt the stressor
- Accept the stressor

Healthy coping styles	Unhealthy coping styles
Exercise	Alcohol or drug use
Having time for self-care	Avoidance of event
Balancing work and play	Procrastination
Proper time management	Overeating

Relaxation Techniques:
- Recognize what activities you consider relaxing.
- Be specific when exploring your options. You might consider the following:
  → Going for walks
  → Meeting with friends
  → Reading for pleasure
  → Listening to music
  → taking a bath
- Begin practicing relaxation techniques like
  → Meditation
  → Deep breathing exercises
  → Progressive relaxation
- Decide which relaxation technique works for you and practice daily.

A-Z of stress management
Following is an action plan to tackle stress:
- Always take time for yourself at least 30 min/day
- Be aware of your own stress meter: Know when to step back and cool down
- Concentrate on controlling your own situation, without controlling everybody else
- Daily exercise will burn off the stress chemicals
- Eat lots of fresh fruit, veggies, bread and water
- Forgive others, do not hold grudges and be tolerant
- Gain perspective on things, how important is the issue
- Have fun and do not be afraid to share your feelings with others
- Identify stressors and plan to deal with them better next time
- Judge your own performance realistically
- Keep a positive attitude
- Limit alcohol, drugs and other stimulant they affect your perception and behavior.
- Manage money well, seek advice and save at least 10% of what you earn
- No is a word you need to learn to use without feeling guilty

- Outdoor activities by yourself or with friends and family, can be a great way to relax.
- Play your favorite music rather than watching television
- Quit smoking
- Relationship: Nurture and enjoy them, learn to listen more and talk less
- Sleep well
- Treat yourself once a week with a massage, dinner out, the movies
- Understand things from the other person's point of view
- Verify information from the source before exploding
- Worry less
- Express: Make a regular retreat to your favorite space, make holidays part of your yearly plan and budget.
- Yearly goal setting: Plan what you want to achieve based on your priorities in your career, relationship, etc.
- Zest for life: Each day is a gift, smile and be thankful that you are a part of the bigger picture.

GRIEF

Experiences of loss are normal and essential in human life. Loss allows a person to change, develop and fulfill his or her innate human potential. Loss may be planned, expected or sudden. Although it can be difficult, loss sometimes is beneficial.

'Grief' refers to the subjective emotions and affect that are a normal response to the experience of loss. Grieving also known as 'bereavement' refers to the process by which a person experiences the grief.

All people grieve when they experience life's changes and losses. 'Anticipatory grieving' is when people facing an expected loss in near future. ' Mourning' is the outward expression of grief.

Types of Losses

If the human needs are unmet, individual experiences loss. They are:
1. Physiological loss
2. Safety loss
3. Loss of security and sense of belonging
4. Loss of self-esteem
5. Loss related to self-actualization.

Grief Reaction

Period	Features
First hour to days	Shock and disbelief, denial of loss, feeling of numbness
Up to	Full awareness of the reality, preoccupation with the loss, anger

6 Months	and resentment over the loss, sadness, guilt, shame, feeling of helplessness, hopelessness and emptiness, sleep disturbance, loss of interest, poor appetite, difficulty in social interactions.
6 Months to 1 year	Restoration of normal functioning and behavior acceptance of reality reappearance of features of the first two phases is possible.

The Grieving Process

For effective nursing interaction with the client, the nurses must have a basic understanding of grieving process. By understanding the process nurses can promote the expression and release of emotions in each stages.

Theory of Grief

Kubler Ross's stages of grieving.

Elizabeth Kubler Ross (1969) established a basis for understanding how losses affects human life. She have attended to clients with terminal illness, she identified five stages of feelings and behavior which people experience as they grieve.

1. Denial: It is a stage of shock and disbelief. It is an immediate response to a loss.
2. Anger: It may be expressed towards God, friends, relatives and health care providers.
3. Bargaining: It occurs when the person asks God or fate for more time to delay the inevitable loss.
   Example: Person may bargain 'If I get cure, I will give money to church'.
4. Depression: Depression results when awareness of the loss becomes acute.
5. Acceptance: The final stage brings a feeling of peace regarding the loss that has occurred. Focus is on the reality of the loss.

Phases or a stage of grief is again explained by Rodebaugh, Schwindt and Valentine in 1999. According to them the process of grief is a journey through four stages:

1. Reeling: The person feels shock, disbelief and denial.
2. Feeling: The person experiences anguish guilt, profound sadness, anger, lack of concentration, sleep disturbances, appetite changes, fatigue and general physical discomfort.
3. Dealing: The person begins to adapt to the loss by engaging in support groups, grief therapy, reading and spiritual guidance.
4. Healing: The person integrates the loss as part of life. The person has accepted the loss.

Resolution is the process in which the person is looking back to loss and association with the lost thing. People accept the pleasure and the disappointments of the association. The person may replace the lost entity with new relationships.

Resolution process may take time if the relationship with the lost entity had been marked by ambivalence, reaction to the loss may be burdened with guilt which lengthens the grief reaction.

If the loss is anticipated, individuals already begins the grieving process before the actual loss. The individual use this time to prepare for the resolution process.

The number of recent losses can affect the resolution process. It become lengthy when a loss occur before complete previous grieving process.

Grief Responses

People have many varied responses to loss. They express their grief in their thoughts, feelings and actions as well as their physiologic responses.

1. *Cognitive responses:* Grieving often causes a person to change beliefs about self and the world. There may be changes in thinking and attitude include reviewing and ranking values, becoming wiser, shedding, illusions about immortality, viewing the world more realistically and re-evaluating religious or spiritual beliefs. Questioning may help the person to accept reality. There may be an attempt to keep the lost one present. For example, there may be a conversation with the died spouse.
2. *Emotional response*: Anger, sadness and anxiety are the predominant emotional responses to loss. Responses also follows the sages of grief.
3. *Spiritual responses*: The personal values embedded in each person give meaning and purpose to life. This values and beliefs are the central components of spirituality and the spiritual responses to grief. The grieving person may angry with God or other religious figures. The anguish behavior loss of hope and loss of meaning can cause deep spiritual suffering.
4. *Behavioral response:* It is easy to observe the behavioral response. Tearfully sobbing, crying uncontrollably, showing restlessness are some of the behavioral response. They may show irritability and hostility towards others. Developing maladaptive responses like drug and alcohol abuse are some of the problems resulting from the grief process. Suicide and homicide attempts may be extreme response. If the bereaved person cannot move through the grieving process. Behavioral responses also follows the stages of grief reaction.
5. *Physiologic responses*: Physiologic symptoms and problems are commonly associated with grieving process. Those grieving may complain of insomnia, headaches, impaired appetite, weight loss, lack of energy, palpitation, indigestion and changes in immune and endocrine systems. Among this sleep disturbance is the most common bereavement symptom.
6. *Maladaptive grief responses:* Maladaptive grief responses to loss occur when an individual is not able to satisfactorily progress through the stages of grieving to achieve resolution.

    These responses are prolonged, delayed/inhibited and distorted responses.
7. *Prolonged responses*: It is characterized by an intense preoccupation with memories of the lost entity for many years after the loss has occurred.

8. *Delayed or inhibited response*: The individual may fixed in denial stage. The person may remain in denial stage until another unrelated loss occur or the same response is triggered by a reminder.
9. *Distorted response*: The individual may fixed in the anger stage of grieving. The normal behaviors associated with grieving such as helplessness, hopelessness, sadness, anger and guilt are exaggerated out of proportion to the situation. This may alter the normal way of functioning. Depression is a distorted grief response.

Treatment

Normal grief does not require any treatment. Complicated grief process requires medication. Nursing interventions are helpful in grieving process rather than medication.

CRISIS

A crisis is a turning point in an individual's life that produces an overwhelming emotional response. Individuals experiences crisis when they face a life circumstance or stress that they cannot manage with their coping skills effectively. Crisis is described as self-limiting; that is the crisis does not last indefinitely at usually exists for 4–6 weeks.

At the end of a period of time, crisis may resolved and person may return to precrisis level of functions or begins to function at the higher level. These are positive outcome. The negative outcome is the person's functioning stabilizes at the level lower than precrisis functioning.

Definition

Crisis is a state of disequilibrium resulting from the interaction of an event with the individual's of family's coping mechanisms, which are inadequate to meet the demands of the situation combined with the individual's of family's perception of the meaning of the event.

Hendricks (1985) suggest that there are some individuals prone to crisis. The risk group are:
- Dissatisfaction with employment or lack of employment
- History of unresolved crisis
- History of substance abuse
- Poor self esteem, unworthiness
- Poor interpersonal relationships
- Difficulty in coping with everyday situations
- Lack of resources and support to manage
- Lack of caring.

Types of Crisis

1. *Maturational crisis*: Maturational crisis is also called developmental crisis. It is associated with normal growth and development and ultimate goal of this

process is called maturity. There are some transition points where individuals move into successive stage which often generate disequilibrium. There are some tasks have to overcome in all stages of development. When an individual fails to meet the task sucessfuly, crisis arise.

The events which is having more crisis potential are adolescence, puberty, marriage, parenthood, menopause, etc.

2. *Situational crisis*: A situational crisis is one that is precipitated by an unanticipated or sudden stressful event. Examples are death of loved one, loss of a job, divorce, etc.
3. *Social crisis*: It is also called adventitious crisis. Social crisis is accidental and unanticipated, results in multiple losses and radical environmental changes. Social crisis includes natural disasters like floods, earthquakes, war, terrorist attacks, contamination of large areas by toxic wastes. The severity and effects of social crisis are more. Support systems may be unavailable because they may also be involved in some crisis.

Phase of Crisis

Caplan (1964) has described phases of crisis.

Phase I

The person is exposed to a stressor, experiences anxiety and tries to cope in a customary fashion.

Phase II

Anxiety arises when customary coping skills are ineffective. The individual experiences a sense of vulnerability.

Phase III

The person makes all possible efforts to deal with the stressor including attempts at new methods of coping. Return to precrisis level of functioning may occur. If problem solving is unsuccessful, further disorganization occurs.

Phase IV

When coping attempts fail, the person experiences disequilibrium and significant distress. Treatment is required.

Signs and Symptoms of Crisis

- Anxiety
- Depression
- Anger and guilt
- Self-care deficit
- Phobia.

Resolution of Crisis

Healthy resolution of a crisis depends on 3 factors:
1. The individual's perception of the event
2. Availability of emotional support
3. Availability of adequate coping mechanisms

The individual may resolve crisis in 3 ways.
1. *Pseudoresolution*: In this, the individual pushes the feelings associated to a crisis out of consciousness. So there will not be any changes in functioning. But in future, when a new crisis arise, it is difficult to resolve the new one as the previous crisis is neither expressed nor handled at the time.
2. *Unsuccessful resolution*: The victim may adapt traditional coping mechanism. But it may not be unsuccessful. The outcome will be negative. The individual may go to a level lower than precrisis level.
3. *Successful resolution*: Victim may go through the phases of crisis, reaches phases IV where various coping measures are utilized and resolution takes place in a positive way. The individual develops skills and problem solving ability. This will help the individual to face a new situation effectively.

Crisis Intervention

Crisis intervention is a technique used to help an individual or family to understand and cope with the intense feelings of crisis. Resolution ends in positive or negative outcomes. Crisis intervention aims at positive outcome. Resolution is influenced by 3 factors, i.e. perception of the event; availability of the emotional support and the availability of adequate coping mechanisms. When a person seeks assistance, these three factors represent a guide for effective intervention. Intervention includes assisting the person to use existing supports or helping the individual to find new sources of support and to learn new methods of coping. Early intervention is associated with better outcomes.

Person experiencing a crisis usually are distressed and likely to seek help for their distress. They are ready to learn and will try new coping skills to resolve the distress. This is an ideal time for intervention and resolution will be successful in terms of positive outcomes.

Types of Intervention

Hemingway, Ashmore and askoorum (2000) identified 2 categories of crisis intervention.
1. *Authoritative interventions*: They are designed to assess the personal health status and promote problem solving such as offering the person new information, knowledge or meaning raising the person's self-awareness by providing feedback about behavior and directing the persons behavior by offering suggestions.
2. *Facilitative interventions*: Facilitative interventions aim at dealing with the person's need for empathetic understanding such as encouraging the person, to identify and discuss feelings and thus facilitates person's self-worth.

Gold Fried states seven steps in crisis intervention:
- Identify the problem
- Propose alternative solutions
- Rehearse each alternative
- Choose one solution

- Define the needed steps
- Take up the steps
- Check the result.

Crisis Intervention Modes

Telephone counseling, home crisis visit, crisis counseling
Common crisis situation:
Insomnia, nightmares, amnesia, social isolation, spiritual distress, anxiety, anger, guilt, hallucination, illusions, potential for violence, rape trauma syndrome.

Appendices

Appendix—1

Common Defense Mechanism

Repression: It is involuntarily forgetting about unacceptable ideas, impulses or events.

Regression: It is immature way of responding to a stress. The individual return a childish form the behavior when faced with a distressing situation to relieve anxiety.

Reaction formation: It is unconscious dealing with unacceptable desires by behaving in opposite way to true feelings.

Projection: Unconsciously shifting the blame on to other people or circumstances.

Rationalizations: It is the joy and delight of the average human being. It is simply finding a logical reason for the things one wants to do.

Intellectualization: Focusing of attention on technical or logical aspects of a threatening situation.

Displacement: It is the transfer of an emotion from its original object to a substitute object.

Sublimation: Primitive impulses are transferred or directed to a socially useful goal. Unacceptable desires find an acceptable outlet.

Identifications: The individual feels the personal satisfaction in the success and achievements of other people and group.

Compensation: It means something given to replace a loss or to make up for a defect.

Denial: The individual does not accept the existence of something that is disturbing.

Suppression: Suppression is an intentional pushing away from awareness of certain unwelcome idea, memories or feelings.

Conversion: Strong emotional conflicts are expressed as or converted into physical symptoms.

Dissociation: Unconsciously removing painful experiences from the conscious mind.

Appendix—2

Common Phobia

Ablutophobia—Fear of washing or bathing.
Achluophobia—Fear of darkness.
Acousticophobia—Fear of noise.
Aeroacrophobia—Fear of open high place.
Aichmophobia—Fear of needles or pointed objects.
Albuminurophobia—Fear of kidney disease.
Alektorophobia—Fear of chickens.
Algophobia—Fear of pain.
Altophobia—Fear of heights.
Amaxophobia—Fear of riding in a car.
Ambulophobia—Fear of walking.
Amnesiphobia—Fear of amnesia.
Amychophobia—Fear of scratches or being scratched.
Androphobia—Fear of men.
Angrophobia—Fear of anger or of becoming angry.
Anthropophobia—Fear of people or society.
Arachnephobia or Arachnophobia—Fear of spiders.
Arsonphobia—Fear of fire.
Atelophobia—Fear of imperfection.
Athazagoraphobia—Fear of being forgotton or ignored or forgetting.
Autophobia—Fear of being alone or of oneself.
Aviophobia or Aviatophobia—Fear of flying

Bacillophobia—Fear of microbes.
Bacteriophobia—Fear of bacteria.
Bibliophobia—Fear of books.
Blennophobia—Fear of slime.
Bromidrosiphobia or Bromidrophobia—Fear of body smells.

Cathisophobia—Fear of sitting.
Catoptrophobia—Fear of mirrors.
Chaetophobia—Fear of hair.
Chorophobia—Fear of dancing.
Cleptophobia—Fear of stealing.
Climacophobia—Fear of stairs, climbing, or of falling downstairs.
Clinophobia—Fear of going to bed.
Coitophobia—Fear of coitus.
Cyberphobia—Fear of computers or working on a computer.

Cyclophobia—Fear of bicycles.
Cynophobia—Fear of dogs or rabies.
Cypridophobia—Fear of prostitutes or venereal disease
Decidophobia—Fear of making decisions.
Dendrophobia—Fear of trees.
Didaskaleinophobia—Fear of going to school.
Dikephobia—Fear of justice.
Dipsophobia—Fear of drinking.
Dromophobia—Fear of crossing streets.
Dystychiphobia—Fear of accidents.

Ecclesiophobia—Fear of church.
Ecophobia—Fear of home.
Electrophobia—Fear of electricity.
Ephebiphobia—Fear of teenagers.
Ergophobia—Fear of work.
Erotophobia—Fear of sexual love or sexual questions.
Galeophobia or Gatophobia—Fear of cats.
Gamophobia—Fear of marriage.
Geliophobia—Fear of laughter.
Gelotophobia—Fear of being laughed at
Glossophobia—Fear of speaking in public or of trying to speak.
Graphophobia—Fear of writing or handwriting.

Haphephobia or Haptephobia—Fear of being touched.
Hedonophobia—Fear of feeling pleasure.
Heliophobia—Fear of the sun.
Hemophobia or Hemaphobia or Hematophobia—Fear of blood.
Heterophobia—Fear of the opposite sex. (Sexophobia)
Hydrophobia—Fear of water or of rabies.
Hypengyophobia or Hypegiaphobia—Fear of responsibility.
Hypnophobia—Fear of sleep or of being hypnotized.

Iatrophobia—Fear of going to the doctor or of doctors.
Iophobia—Fear of poison.

Kleptophobia—Fear of stealing
Kolpophobia—Fear of genitals, particularly female.

Lachanophobia—Fear of vegetables.
Laliophobia or Lalophobia—Fear of speaking
Logophobia—Fear of words.
Lygophobia—Fear of darkness.
Mageirocophobia—Fear of cooking.
Mastigophobia—Fear of punishment.
Mechanophobia—Fear of machines.

Menophobia—Fear of menstruation.
Metathesiophobia—Fear of changes.
Methyphobia—Fear of alcohol.
Misophobia or Mysophobia—Fear of being contaminated with dirt or germs.
Mnemophobia—Fear of memories.
Motorphobia—Fear of automobiles.

Necrophobia—Fear of death or dead things.
Nelophobia—Fear of glass.
Neopharmaphobia—Fear of new drugs.
Neophobia—Fear of anything new.
Noctiphobia—Fear of the night.
Nosocomephobia—Fear of hospitals.
Ochlophobia—Fear of crowds or mobs.
Odontophobi— Fear of teeth or dental surgery.
Olfactophobia—Fear of smells.
Ombrophobia—Fear of rain or of being rained on.
Oneirophobia—Fear of dreams.

Paralipophobia—Fear of neglecting duty or responsibility.
Parthenophobia—Fear of virgins or young girls.
Pathophobia—Fear of disease.
Parturiphobia—Fear of childbirth.
Pedophobia—Fear of children.
Peniaphobia—Fear of poverty.
Pentheraphobia—Fear of mother-in-law. (Novercaphobia)
Pharmacophobia—Fear of taking medicine.
Philemaphobia or Philematophobia—Fear of kissing.
Philophobia—Fear of falling in love or being in love.
Photophobia—Fear of light.
Potamophobia—Fear of rivers or running water.
Potophobia—Fear of alcohol.
Psychrophobia—Fear of cold.
Pyrexiophobia—Fear of Fever.

Radiophobia—Fear of radiation, X-rays.
Rhypophobia—Fear of defecation.
Rhytiphobia—Fear of getting wrinkles.
Rupophobia—Fear of dirt.

Scriptophobia—Fear of writing in public.
Selenophobia—Fear of the moon.
Sesquipedalophobia—Fear of long words.
Siderodromophobia—Fear of trains, railroads or train travel.
Itophobia or Sitiophobia—Fear of food or eating. (Cibophobia)
Somniphobia—Fear of sleep.

Stasibasiphobia or Stasiphobia—Fear of standing or walking. (Ambulophobia)
Syngenesophobia—Fear of relatives.

Technophobia—Fear of technology.
Telephonophobia—Fear of telephones.
Thaasophobia—Fear of sitting.
Thalassophobia—Fear of the sea.
Theophobia—Fear of gods or religion.
Tomophobia—Fear of surgical operations.
Traumatophobia—Fear of injury.
Trichopathophobia or Trichophobia—Fear of hair. (Chaetophobia, Hypertrichophobia)
Trypanophobia—Fear of injections.

Uranophobia or Ouranophobia—Fear of heaven.
Urophobia—Fear of urine or urinating.

Venustraphobia—Fear of beautiful women.
Verbophobia—Fear of words.
Verminophobia—Fear of germs.
Vestiphobia—Fear of clothing.
Virginitiphobia—Fear of rape.

Xenoglossophobia—Fear of foreign languages.
Xenophobia—Fear of strangers or foreigners.
Xerophobia—Fear of dryness.

Zelophobia—Fear of jealousy.
Zoophobia—Fear of animals.

Appendix—3

Manias

Ablutomania	mania for washing oneself
Aboulomania	pathological indecisiveness
Agromania	intense desire to be in open spaces
Andromania	nymphomania
Anglomania	craze or obsession with England and the English
Anthomania	obsession with flowers
Aphrodisiomania	abnormal sexual interest
Arithmomania	obsessive preoccupation with numbers
Balletomania	abnormal fondness for ballet
Bibliomania	craze for books or reading
Bruxomania	compulsion for grinding teeth
Cacodemomania	pathological belief that one is inhabited by an evil spirit
Catapedamania	obsession with jumping from high places
Chinamania	obsession with collecting china
Choreomania	dancing mania or frenzy
Clinomania	excessive desire to stay in bed
Copromania	obsession with feces
Cytheromania	nymphomania
Dacnomania	obsession with killing
Demonomania	pathological belief that one is possessed by demons
Dinomania	mania for dancing
Dipsomania	abnormal craving for alcohol
Discomania	obsession for disco music
Doramania	obsession with owning furs
Doromania	obsession with giving gifts
Drapetomania	intense desire to run away from home
Dromomania	compulsive longing for travel
Ecdemomania	abnormal compulsion for wandering
Egomania	irrational self-centered attitude or self-worship
Eleutheromania	manic desire for freedom
Empleomania	mania for holding public office

Enosimania	pathological belief that one has sinned
Entheomania	abnormal belief that one is divinely inspired
Epomania	craze for writing epics
Ergasiomania	excessive desire to work; ergomania
Ergomania	excessive desire to work; workaholism
Erotomania	abnormally powerful sex drive
Etheromania	craving for ether
Ethnomania	obsessive devotion to one's own people
Eulogomania	obsessive craze for eulogies
Flagellomania	abnormal enthusiasm for flogging
Florimania	craze for flowers
Francomania	craze or obsession with France and the French
Gallomania	craze or obsession with France and the French
Gamomania	obsession with issuing odd marriage proposals
Grecomania	obsession with Greece and the Greeks
Graphomania	obsession with writing
Gynecomania	abnormal sexual obsession with women
Habromania	insanity featuring cheerful delusions
Hagiomania	mania for sainthood
Hellenomania	obsession with Greece and the Greeks; Grecomania
Hexametromania	mania for writing in hexameter
Hieromania	pathological religious visions or delusions
Hippomania	obsession with horses
Hydromania	irrational craving for water
Hylomania	excessive tendency towards materialism
Hypermania	severe mania
Hypomania	minor mania
Hysteromania	nymphomania
Iconomania	obsession with icons or portraits
Idolomania	obsession or devotion to idols
Infomania	excessive devotion to accumulating facts
Islomania	craze or obsession for islands
Italomania	obsession with Italy or Italians
Kleptomania	irrational predilection for stealing
Klopemania	kleptomania
Logomania	pathological loquacity
Lypemania	extreme pathological mournfulness
Macromania	delusion that objects are larger than natural size
Megalomania	abnormal tendency towards grand or grandiose behavior

Melomania	craze for music
Methomania	morbid craving for alcohol
Metromania	insatiable desire for writing verse
Micromania	pathological self-deprecation or belief that one is very small
Monomania	abnormal obsession with a single thought or idea
Morphinomania	habitual craving or desire for morphine
Musomania	obsession with music
Mythomania	lying or exaggerating to an abnormal extent
Narcomania	uncontrollable craving for narcotics
Necromania	sexual obsession with dead bodies; necrophilia
Nosomania	delusion of suffering from a disease
Nostomania	abnormal desire to go back to familiar places
Nymphomania	excessive or crazed sexual desire
Oenomania	obsession or craze for wine
Oligomania	obsession with a few thoughts or ideas
Oniomania	mania for making purchases
Onomamania	mania for names
Onomatomania	irresistible desire to repeat certain words
Onychotillomania	compulsive picking at the fingernails
Opiomania	craving for opium
Opsomania	abnormal love for one kind of food
Orchidomania	abnormal obsession with orchids
Palermomania	mania for war
Parousiamania	obsession with the second coming of Christ
Pathomania	moral insanity
Peotillomania	abnormal compulsion for pulling on the penis
Phagomania	excessive desire for food or eating
Phaneromania	habit of biting one's nails
Pharmacomania	abnormal obsession with trying drugs
Phonomania	pathological tendency to murder
Photomania	pathological desire for light
Phyllomania	excessive or abnormal production of leaves
Phytomania	obsession with collecting plants
Planomania	abnormal desire to wander and disobey social norms
Plutomania	mania for money
Politicomania	mania for politics
Polkamania	craze for polka dancing
Polymania	mania affecting several different mental faculties
Poriomania	abnormal compulsion to wander

Pornomania	obsession with pornography
Potichomania	craze for imitating oriental porcelain
Potomania	abnormal desire to drink alcohol
Pseudomania	irrational predilection for lying
Pteridomania	passion for ferns
Pyromania	craze for starting fires
Rhinotillexomania	compulsive nose picking
Rinkomania	obsession with skating
Satyromania	abnormally great male sexual desire; satyriasis
Scribbleomania	obsession with scribbling
Sebastomania	religious insanity
Sitiomania	morbid aversion to food
Sophomania	delusion that one is incredibly intelligent
Squandermania	irrational propensity for spending money wastefully
Stampomania	obsession with stamp-collecting
Syphilomania	pathological belief that one is afflicted with syphilis
Technomania	craze for technology
Teutomania	obsession with Teutonic or German things
Thanatomania	belief that one has been affected by death magic, and resulting illness
Theatromania	craze for going to plays
Theomania	belief that one is a god
Timbromania	craze for stamp collecting
Tomomania	irrational predilection for performing surgery
Toxicomania	morbid craving for poisons
Trichotillomania	neurosis where patient pulls out own hair
Tulipomania	obsession with tulips
Typhomania	delirious state resulting from typhus fever
Typomania	craze for printing one's lucubrations
Uranomania	obsession with the idea of divinity
Verbomania	craze for words
Xenomania	inordinate attachment to foreign things
Zoomania	insane fondness for animals.

Appendix—4

Paraphilias

Abasiophilia: Love of (or sexual attraction to) people who use leg braces or other orthopedic appliances.

Acousticophilia: Sexual arousal from certain sounds.

Agalmatophilia: Sexual attraction to statues or mannequins or immobility.

Algolagnia: Sexual pleasure from pain.

Amaurophilia: Sexual arousal by a partner whom one is unable to see due to artificial means, such as being blindfolded or having sex in total darkness (see: sensory deprivation).

Andromimetophilia: Love of women dressed as men.

Apodysophilia: Desire to undress, see also nudism.

Apotemnophilia: Desire to have (or sexual arousal from having) a healthy appendage (limb, digit, or male genitals) amputated.

Aquaphilia: Arousal from water and/or in watery environments, including bathtubs or swimming pools.

Aretifism: Sexual attraction to people who are without footwear, in contrast to retifism.

Asphyxiophilia: Sexual attraction to asphyxia; also called breath control play; including autoerotic asphyxiation; see medical warnings.

Autogynephilia: Love of oneself as a woman (also see Blanchard, Bailey, and Lawrence theory for discussion on controversy).

Biastophilia: Sexual pleasure from committing rape.

Celebriphilia: Pathological desire to have sex with a celebrity.

Coprophilia: Sexual attraction to (or pleasure from) feces.

Crush fetish: Sexual arousal from seeing small creatures being crushed by members of the opposite sex, or being crushed oneself.

Dacryphilia: Sexual pleasure in eliciting tears from others or oneself.

Dendrophilia: Sexual attraction to trees and other large plants, popularized by the movie "Superstar" with Molly Shannon.

Diaper fetishism: Sexual arousal from diapers.

Emetophilia (a.k.a. vomerophilia): Sexual attraction to vomit.

Ephebophilia (a.k.a. hebephilia): Sexual attraction towards adolescents.

Eproctophilia: Sexual attraction to flatulence.

Exhibitionism: Sexual arousal through sexual behavior in view of third parties (also includes the recurrent urge or behavior to expose one's genitals to an unsuspecting person, known as indecent exposure).

Faunoiphilia: Sexual arousal from watching animals mate.

Fetishism: It is the use of non-sexual or nonliving objects or part of a person's body to gain sexual excitement. Examples include: Balloon fetishism—breast fetishism—foot fetishism (podophilia)—fur fetishism—leather fetishism—lipstick fetishism—medical fetishism—panty fetishism—robot fetishism—rubber fetishism—shoe fetishism—smoking fetishism—spandex fetishism—dental braces fetishism—transvestic fetishism (see below).

Frotteurism: Sexual arousal from the recurrent urge or behavior of touching or rubbing against a nonconsenting person.

Galactophilia: Sexual attraction to human milk or lactating women (incorrect term).

Gerontophilia: Sexual attraction towards the elderly.

Hematophilia: Sexual attraction involving blood (either on a sex partner/attractive person or the liquid itself; not to be confused with hemophilia, a genetic disorder of the blood).

Harpaxophilia: Sexual arousal from being the victim of a robbery or burglary.

Hematolagnia: Sexual attraction to blood.

Hybristophilia: Sexual arousal to people who have committed crimes, in particular cruel or outrageous crimes.

Infantilism: Sexual pleasure from dressing, acting, or being treated as a baby.

Katoptronophilia: Sexual arousal from having sex in front of mirrors.

Klismaphilia: Sexual pleasure from enemas.

Lust murder: Sexual arousal through committing murder.

Macrophilia: Sexual attraction to larger people and large things (including larger body organs such as breasts and genitalia).

Maiesiophilia: Sexual attraction to childbirth or pregnant women.

Masochism: It is the recurrent urge or behavior of wanting to be humiliated, beaten, bound, or otherwise made to suffer.

Microphilia: Sexual attraction to smaller people and things of smaller size.

Mysophilia: Sexual attraction to soiled, dirty, foul or decaying material.

Necrophilia: Sexual attraction to corpses.

Necrozoophilia: Sexual attraction to the corpses or killings of animals (also known as necrobestiality).

Nepiophilia: The same as infantophilia sexual attraction to children between the age of 0–3 years.

Pedophilia: Sexual attraction to prepubescent children (British spelling: paedophilia).

Phalloorchoalgolagnia: Sexual arousal by the experiencing of painful stimuli being administered to the male genitals.

Pictophilia: Sexual attraction to pictorial pornography/erotic art.

Plushophilia: Sexual attraction to stuffed toys or people in animal costume, such as theme park characters.

Pyrophilia: Sexual arousal through watching, setting, hearing/talking/fantasizing about fire.

Retifism: Sexual arousal from shoes.

Sadism: Sexual arousal from giving pain.

Schediaphilia (aka Toonophilia): Love (or sexual arousal) to cartoon characters/situations.

Sitophilia: Sexual arousal from food.

Somnophilia: Sexual arousal from sleeping or unconscious people.

Spectrophilia: Sexual attraction to ghosts.

Telephone scatologia: Being sexually aroused by making obscene telephone calls.

Teratophilia: Sexual attraction to deformed or monstrous people.

Transformation fetish: Sexual arousal from depictions of transformations of people into objects or other beings.

Transvestic fetishism: It is a sexual attraction towards the clothing of the opposite gender (also known as transvestitism).

Trichophilia: Love (or sexual arousal) from hair.

Urolagnia: Sexual attraction to urine.

Vorarephilia: Sexual attraction to being eaten by, and/or eating, another person or creature.

Voyeurism: Sexual arousal through watching others having sex (also includes the recurrent urge or behavior to observe an unsuspecting person who is naked, disrobing or engaging in sexual activities, see peeping tom).

Xenophilia: Sexual attraction to foreigners (in science fiction, can also mean sexual attraction to aliens).

Zoophilia: Emotional or sexual attraction to animals.

Zoosadism: The sexual enjoyment of causing pain and suffering to animals.

Glossary

A

Abnormal behavior: It describes a person's covert and overt activities that are deviating from the normal behavior.

Abreaction: Emotional release or discharge after recalling a painful experience.

Addictiction: The biological and/or psychosocial behaviors related to substance dependence.

Adiadochokinesia: Inability to perform rapid alternating movement.

Affect: Observed expression of emotion.

Aggression: Forceful goal directed action that may be verbal or physical.

Agitation: Severe anxiety associated with motor restlessness.

Agnosia: Inability to recognized and interpret the significance of sensory impression.

Alexithymia: Inability or difficulty in describing or being aware of one's emotion or mood.

Ambivalence: Coexistence of two opposing impulses towards the same thing in the same person at the same time.

Amnesia: Partial or total inability to recall past experiences.

Anhedonia: Inability to experience pleasure in any activity.

Anosognosia: Ignorance of illness.

Anterograde amnesia: Amnesia for events occurring after a point in time.

Anxiety: Anxiety is the subjective emotional response to the stressor.

Anxiety amnesia: Lack of memory due to morbid anxiety.

Apathy: Lack of feeling, interest or emotion.

Aphasia: Disutility findings the right word.

Appropriate affect: Condition in which the emotional tone is in harmony with the accompanying idea, thought or speech.

Apraxia: Inability to carryout specific tasks.

Astereognosis: Inability to recognize objects by touch.

Attention: The ability to focus on one activity in a sustained, concentrated manner.

Ataxia: Failure of muscle coordination.

Auditory hallucination: False perception of sound as voice, noise, music, etc.

B

Behavior: Behavior means all the covert and overt activities of human being that can be observed.

Blunted affect: A disturbance in affect manifested by a severe reduction in the intensity of externalized feeling tone.

Bisexuality: A sexual attraction to people of both sexes and the engagement in both homosexual and heterosexual activity.

C

Cataplexy: Temporary loss of muscle tone and weakness precipitated by a variety of emotional states.

Catalepsy: General term for an immobile position that is constantly maintained.

Catatonic excitement: Agitates, purposeless motor activity, uninfluenced by external stimuli.

Catatonic rigidity: Voluntary assumption of a rigid posture, held against all efforts to be moved.

Catatonic stupor: Markedly slowed motor activity and seeming unawareness or surroundings.

Catatonic posturing: Voluntary assumption of an inappropriate posture, generally maintained for long period of time.

Catharsis: Release that occurs when the patient is encouraged to talk about things that bother him or her most. Fears, feelings and experiences are brought out into the open and discussed.

Circumstantiality: Indirect speech that in delayed in reaching the point but eventually gets from original point to desired goal.

Clouding of consciousness: Incomplete clear-mindedness with disturbances in perception and attitudes.

Cognition: The mental process characterized by knowing, thinking, learning and judging.

Conflict: Clashing of two opposing interests. The person experiences two competing drives and must choose between them.

Coma: Profound degree of unconsciousness.

Compulsion: Repetitive stereotyped act performed to relieve fear connected with obsession.

Coprolalia: Compulsive utterance of obscene words.

Condensation: Fusion of various concepts into one.

Clang association: Association of words similar in sound but not in meaning

D

Decision making: Arriving at a solution or making a choice.

Delinquency: A minor violation of legal or moral codes, especially by children or adolescents.

Delusion: False unshakable belief.

Delusion of control: False feeling that one's will, thought or feelings are being controlled by external forces.

Delusion of grandeur: An individual's belief that he is somebody special has some special power, ability, wealth or status.

Delusion of persecutions: An individual's belief that other persons, groups or people are out to harm in some way.

Delusion of reference: An individual may falsely believe that other are talking about him.

Delusion of control: This refers to the belief that the patient's will, thought or feelings are being controlled by external forces.

Delusion of infidelity (delusion of jealousy): This is the delusion that one's lover is unfaithful to him/her.

Delusion of guilt: Belief that one in a sinner and is responsible for the ruin of his family or society.

Depersonalization disorder: A dissociative disorder characterized by intense, prolonged, or otherwise troubling feelings of detachment from one's body or thoughts, not secondary to another mental disorder.

Depression: Psychopathological feeling of sadness.

Diurnal variation: Mood is regularly worst in the morning immediately after awakening, and improver as the day progresses.

Disruptive behavior disorders: A group of mental disorders of children and adolescents consisting of behavior that violates social norms and is disruptive.

Disorientation: Disturbance of orientation in time, place or person.

Distractibility: Inability to concentrate attention.

Dysphoric mood: An unplanned mood.

Dysprosody: Loss of normal speech melody.

Dysarthria: Difficulty in articulation, not in word finding or in grammar.

E

Echolalia: Psychopathological repeating of words or phrases of one person by another.

Echopraxia: Pathological imitation of movements of one person by another.

Ecstasy: Feeling of intense rapture.

Egomania: Pathological self-preoccupation.

Elevated mood: A mood more cheerful than usual.

Erotomania: Delusional belief, more common in women than in men, that someone in deeply in love with them.

Euthymic mood: Normal range of mood.

Euphoria: Increased sense or psychological well being and happiness not in keeping with ongoing events.

Expansive mood: Expression of one's feelings without restraint.

Exogenous: Developing or originating outside the organism.

F

Fear: Fear involves the intellectual appraisal of a threatening stimulus.

Flat affect: Absence or near absence of any signs of affective expression.

Flight of ideas: Rapid, continuous on words produce constant shifting from one idea to another in logical way.

G

Grief: Sadness appropriate to a real loss.

Guilt: Emotion secondary to doing what is perceived as wrong.

Gustatory hallucination: False perception of taste.

H

Hallucination: False sensory perception in the absence of external stimuli.

Hallucinosis: Hallucination that is associated with chronic alcohol abuse.

Health: Health is a state of complete physical, mental and social well being and not merely the absent of disease or infirmity.

Heterosexuality: Sexual attraction to members of the opposite sex.

Homosexuality: sexual attraction to members of the same sex.

Hypervigilance: Excessive attention and focus on all internal and external stimuli, usually secondary to delusional or paranoid states.

Hypnagogic hallucination: False sensory perception occurring while falling sleep.

Hypnopompic hallucination: False sensory perception occurring which awakening from sleep.

I

Inappropriate affect: Disharmony between the emotional feeling tone and the idea, thought or speech accompanying it.

Insight: Ability of the patient to understand the true cause and meaning of a situation.

Irritable mood: Easily annoyed and provoked to anger.

Illusion: Misperception of real external sensory stimuli.

Incoherence: Thought that is not understandable resulting in disorganization.

J

Judgment: Ability to assess a situation correctly and to act appropriately within that situation.

L

Labile affect: Rapid and abrupt changer in emotional feeling tone, untreated to external stimuli.

Lethologica: Temporary inability to remember a name or a proper noun.

Lilliputian hallucination: False perception in which objects are seen as reduced in size.

Logorrhea: Excessive uncontrolled speech.

Loosening of associations: Flow of thought in which idea shift from one subject to another in a completely illogical way.

M

Mannerism: Ingrained, habitual involuntary movement.

Mental disorder: Any clinically significant behavioral or psychological syndrome characterized by the presence of distressing symptoms, impairment

of functioning, or significantly increased risk of suffering death, pain, or other disability.

Mental health: Mental health is defined as the capacity of an individual to form harmonious relationship with others and to participate in, or contribute constrictively to, change in the social environment.

Mental Illness: Mental illness occurs when a state of physical, mental and social well being is disturbed.

Moodswings: Oscillation between euphoria and depression or anxiety.

Monomania: Preoccupation with single object.

Motor behavior (Conation): The aspect of the psyche that includes impulses, motivation, wishes, drives and instincts as expressed by a person's behavior or motor activity.

Mutism: Voicelessness without structural abnormalities.

N

Negativism: Motiveless resistance to all attempts to be moved or all instructions.

Neologism: New word created by the patient.

Neurosis: It is a group minor mental disorder. Person suffering from neurosis do not lose touch with reality and they are able to meet the ordinary demands of everyday living. Neurotic people do not cause much trouble to others but they themselves experience varying degrees of personal distress and suffering.

O

Obsession: A mental state where one is occupied with uncontrollable desire, idea or emotion even thought he knows fully about it.

Olfactory hallucination: False perception of smell.

Orgasm: Peaking of sexual pleasure and the release of sexual tension accompanied by rhythmic contraction of the perineal muscles and pelvic reproductive organs.

P

Perseveration: Repetition of meaningless words, phrases or answers.

Phobia: Irrational fear resulting in desire to avoid the feared object/situation.

Pressure of speech: Rapid production of speech output with a subjective feeling of racing thoughts.

Prosopagnisia: Inability to recognize faces.

Poverty of speech: Restriction in the amount of speech used poverty of content of speech: Speech that in adequate in amount but conveys little information because of vagueness or emptiness.

Psychosis: It is a severe type of mental illness in which the patient talks and behaves abnormally. The function of the body and mind are severely disturbed resulting in gross impairment of individual and social activities. He loses touch with reality.

Psychiatric disorder: Psychiatric disorder in a disturbance of cognition (thought) or conation (action) or affect (feeling) or any disequilibrium between the three.

Psychiatric Nursing: Psychiatric nursing is the promotion of mental health, prevention of mental illness and care of rehabilitation of a patient with mental illness.

R

Relapse: Return of symptoms.

Restricted affect: Reduction in intensity of feeling tone less severe than blunted affect but really reduced.

Retrograde amnesia: Amnesia prior to a point in time.

S

Seclusion: Separating the patient from others in a safe, contained environment with minimal stimulation.

Self-esteem: The person's judgement of personal worth obtained by analysis how well his or her behavior conforms to self-ideal.

Selection inattention: Blocking out only those things that generate anxiety.

Somnolence: Abnormal drowsiness.

Somnambulism: Motor activity during sleep.

Somatization disorder: A somatoform disorder characterized by multiple somatic complaints, including a combination of pain, gastrointestinal, sexual, and neurological symptoms, and not fully explainable by any known general medical condition or the direct effect of a substance, but not intentionally feigned or produced.

Somatoform disorders: Mental disorders characterized by symptoms suggesting physical disorders of psychogenic origin but not under voluntary control, e.g. body dysmorphic disorder, conversion disorder, hypochondriasis, pain disorder, somatization disorder, and undifferentiated somatoform disorder.

Somatic delusion: It is concerned with illness. The patient may believe wrongly and in the face of all medical evidence to the contrary that he is ill.

Somatopagnosia: Inability to recognize a body part as one's own.

Stereo type: Constant repetitions especially needless or purposeless activity is called stereotype.

Stupor: Lack of reaction and unaware of surrounding.

Stuttering: Frequent repetition or prolongation of a sound or syllable, leading to markedly impaired speech fluency.

Stigma: An attribute or trait deemed by the person's social environment as negative, different and diminishing.

Sunrise syndrome: Unstable cognitive ability upon rising in the morning.

Sundowning syndrome: Cognitive ability diminishing in the late afternoon or early evening.

Synethesia: Sensation or hallucination caused by another sensation. For example a sound is experienced as being seen, or a visual experience is heard.

T

Tactile hallucination: False perception of touch or surface sensation.

Tangentiality: Inability to have goal directed associations of thought.

Tension: Increased motor and psychological activity that in unpleasant.

Thought block: Sudden interruption of steam of speech or thinking.

Thought withdrawal: Delusion that one's thought are being removed from one's mind by other people or forces.

Thought insertion: Delusion that thought are being implanted in one's mind by other people or forces.

Thought broad casting: Delusion that one's thought can be heard by other, as thought they were being broadcast into the air.

Thought control: Delusion that one's thought are being controlled by other people or forces.

Trance: Focused attention and altered consciousness usually seen in hypnosis and dissociative disorder.

Tic: Involuntary, spasmodic motor movement.

Twilight: Disturbed conscious with hallucination.

V

Verbigeration: Meaningless repetition of specific words or phrases.

Visual hallucination: False perception involving sight consisting of both formed images (people) and unformed images (flashes of light).

Visual agnosia: Inability to recognize objects or persons.

W

Waxy flexibility: Parts of body can be placed in positions that will be maintained for long periods of time, even if very uncomfortable.

Word Salad: Incoherent mixture of words and phrases.

V

Verbigeration: Meaningless repetition of specific words or phrases.

Visual hallucination: False perception involving sight consisting of both formed images (people) and unformed images (flashes of light).

Visual agnosia: Inability to recognize objects or persons.

W

Waxy flexibility: Parts of body can be placed in positions that will be maintained for long periods of time, even if very uncomfortable.

Word Salad: Incoherent mixture of words and phrases.

Index

A

Abstinence 94
Achievement and aptitude tests 38
Acupuncture 202
Acute
   and transient psychotic disorder 72
      treatment 73
   polymorphic psychotic disorder with symptoms of schizophrenia 71
   treatment of manic episodes 64
Advantages of
   classical conditioning techniques 185
   therapeutic community 193
Agoraphobia 78
Alcohol
   use disorder 96
   withdrawal state 68
Alzheimer's disease 69, 71
Analytically oriented sex therapy 139
Anorexia nervosa 114
Anti-anxiety drugs 177
Anti-depressant drugs 176
Anti-manic drugs 175
Anti-psychotic drugs 173
Anti-social personality disorder 130
Anxiety 12, 76, 213, 220
Anxious personality disorder 130
Arousal disorders 125
Asperger syndrome 148
Attention deficit hyperactivity disorder 150
Autism spectrum disorder 148
Autistic disorder 148
Aversion therapy 183

B

Behavior therapy 66, 100, 139
Behavioral
   psychotherapy 160
   theory 76, 82
   therapy 152
Binge eating disorder 116
Biological theory 76, 82
Biopsychosocial therapies 172
Bipolar disorders 62
Bleuler classification of symptoms 56
Borderline personality disorder 214, 221
Brain defects or injury 10
Bulimia nervosa 115
Burden of disease 205

C

Caffeine-related disorder 106
Cancer 68
Cannabis intoxication 106
Capgras syndrome 74
Cardiovascular
   disorders 127
   system 225
Cataplexy 123
Catatonic schizophrenia 55
Causes of
   ADHD 151
   hyperventilation syndrome 89
   mental disorders 9
   mood disorders 59
   psychiatric disturbance 140
Central
   nervous system 4, 67, 107
   sleep apnea syndrome 124
Cerebral palsy 144
Childhood mental disorder 12, 140
Circadian rhythm sleep disorders 125
Citrated calcium carbimide 101
Classical conditioning theory 80
Classification of
   anxiolytes 177
   mental
      disorders 10
      retardation 145
   recreational activities 198
Cocaine
   and related disorder 104
   induced disorders 104
   intoxication 104
   withdrawal 105
Cognitive behavior therapy 66, 185
Colonoscopy 91
Common techniques psychotherapy 179
Communication skills 39
Community mental health 205
Complex motor tics 154
Complications of alcohol dependence 98

Components of
   communication process 39
   history collection 26
   therapeutic community 192
Conduct disorder 156
Conscious mind 18
Context of therapeutic communication 41
Conversion disorder 84
Coping strategy 233
Couples therapy 195
Course of schizophrenia 55
Covert sensitization 184
Cranial nerves 33
Creutzfeldt-Jacob disease 67
Crisis 238
   intervention modes 241
   situation 230
Cyclothymic disorder 62

D

Dangers of binge eating 116
Deep tendon reflexes 37
Degenerative disorders 67
Delirium 68
   and dementia 12
Delusional disorder 73
Delusions 56, 57
Dementia 68
Dependence syndrome 98
Dependent
   personality disorder 130
   reaction transference 49
Depression 12, 213, 220
Depressive
   disorders 60
   episode 60
Desensitization 182
Detoxification 95, 100
Developmental disorders 11
Diabetes 174
Diabulimia 116
Diffuse Lewy body disease 67
Disorders of perception 56
Disorganized
   behavior 57
   schizophrenia 55
Dissociative disorder 85
District Mental Health Program 206
Dizziness 174
Dopamine hypothesis 53
Down syndrome 71, 143
Drug
   abuse 95
   dependence 95

   management of acute mania 64
   misuse 95
Dual sex therapy 138
Dyspareunia 136, 137
Dysthymic disorder 61

E

Early morning awakening 128
Eating disorders 115, 213, 220
Electroconvulsive therapy 199
Electroencephalogram 128
Electronic communications 204
Elements of therapeutic community 192
Elimination disorder 157
Emergency psychiatry 162
Emotion 29
Emotionally unstable personality disorder 131
Encopresis 158
Enuresis 157
Environmental disorder 155
Erectile disorder 139
Erik Erikson's 8 stages of psychosocial development 21
Explaing Johari window 47
Exploitation 24
Extrinsic sleep disorders 125

F

Family
   discord 141
   theories 54
   therapy 59
Female
   orgasmic disorder 136
   sexual arousal disorder 136
Fernic chloride test 143
Food maintenance syndrome 115
Forms of drug 104
Fragile X-syndrome 144
Freud theory 18
Functional psychosis 12, 51

G

Gastrointestinal
   disorders 127
   system 226
General
   adaptation syndrome 231
   adaptation syndrome model 231
   cognitive model 186
Generalized anxiety disorder 77

Golden age of neuropsychiatry 5
Group therapy 66, 139
Guthrie's test 143

H

Habit disorders 153
Head injury 126
Histrionic personality disorder 131
Hormonal imbalances 126
Hormone therapy 138
Hospital acquired sleep disturbances 127
Huntington's disease 67
Hyperphagic short stature 115
Hyperventilation syndrome 89, 166
Hypnagogic hallucinations 123
Hypnotherapy 139
Hypoactive sexual desire disorder 136
Hysteria 12
Hysterical neurosis 84

I

Id, ego, and superego 20
Idiopathic insomnia 123
Indian
    classification of mental disorder 12
    Lunacy Act 167
Inhalant
    intoxication 110
    use disorder 110
Insomnia 123
Integumentary system 224
Intellectual functioning 227
Intelligence tests 38
Interdisciplinary treatment team 13
Interpersonal
    communication 40
    therapy 66
Intrinsic sleep disorders 123
Irritable bowel syndrome 90

J

Jacobson progressive
    muscle relaxation 181
    relational technique 78
Johari window 46

K

Kidney disease 68
Kinds of
    stress 233
    stressors 230

Kohlberg's theory 23
Korsakoff's syndrome 71

L

Lazarus's cognitive appraisal model 231
Legal aspects of psychiatry 167
Lifelong female orgasmic disorder 139
Light therapy 199
Liver disease 68
Lower gastrointestinal series 91
Lysergic acid diethylamide 111

M

Major depressive disorder 60, 61
Male
    erectile disorder 136
    orgasmic disorder 136, 137
Management of
    mixed bipolar disorder 65
    suicidal person 164
Mania and depression 12
Manic episode 59
Marital therapy 195
Master of psychiatric nursing 7
Maturational crisis 238
Memory functioning 226
Mental
    disorders 8
        disorders for special people 212
        in elders 223
        in women 212
    Health
        Act 167
        assessment 26
        care 206
        disorders 212
        emergency care 16
        technician 14
        treatment 202
    illness 148
    retardation 12, 142, 148
    status examination 28
Mild mental retardation 145
Milieu therapy 188, 191
Mini mental status examination 31
Model of stress 231
Moderate mental retardation 145
Modern era of medicine 4
Modified electroconvulsive therapy 199
Monoamine oxidase inhibitors 177
Mood disorders 59, 62
Moral developmental theory 23

Motor
    system 36
    tics 154
Multi-infract dementia 69
Multiple
    sclerosis 67
    sleep latency test 128
Musculoskeletal system 225
Music
    therapist 14
    therapy 196

N

Narcissistic personality disorder 131
Narcolepsy 123
Narcotic 101
    drugs and psychotropic 171
National Mental Health Program 205, 206
Nervous system 223
Neuroleptic malignant syndrome 175
Neuropsychological tests 38
Neurosis 12
Neurotic disorders 76
Neurotransmitter imbalances 126
Nightmares 126
Non-rapid eye movement sleep 121
Nonverbal communication 41
Normal pressure hydrocephalus 68

O

Obesity 119
Obsessive compulsive disorder 12, 81, 213
Obstructive sleep apnea syndrome 124
Occupational
    tests 38
    therapist 14
    therapy 195
Opioid
    abuse 101
    and related disorder 101
    dependence 101, 102
    intoxication 102
    withdrawal 102
Organic
    amnestic syndrome 71
    mental disorders 67
    psychosis 12
Orgasmic disorder 136

P

Pain symptoms 120
Panic disorder 77

Paranoid
    personality disorder 132
    schizophrenia 55
Parasomnias 125, 126
Parkinson's disease 68
Peplau's
    interpersonal theory 23
    theory 23
Perinatal
    disorders 221
    mental disorders 214
Periodic limb movement disorder 124
Personality
    disorders 11, 12, 129
    tests 38
Pervasive developmental disorder 148
Phenylketonuria 143
Phobia 12
Phobic disorder 78
Piaget's theory of cognitive development 24
Pick's disease 68
Polysomnography 128
Post-schizophrenia depression 56
Post-traumatic stress disorder 86, 212
Premature ejaculation 136, 137
Premenstrual
    dysphoria 8
    dysphoric disorder 61
    syndrome 87, 214
Prevalence of mental disorders 7
Primary
    obsessive slowness 83
    snoring 126
Principles of
    dance movement therapy 197
    mental health nursing 12
    milieu therapy 188
Profound mental retardation 145
Psychiatric
    day
        hospital 209
        training center 209
    disorders 126, 142, 143
    emergency 162
    nurse 13
    rehabilitation 208
    revolution 6
    social worker 14
Psychiatry 1
Psychoactive
    drugs 93
    substance use disorder 12, 93
Psychoanalytic psychotherapy 66
Psychoanalytical theories 55

Psychodrama 197
Psychodynamic
  theory 80
  treatment 133
Psychogenic hyperventilation syndrome 89
Psychological
  tests 38
  theories 54
Psychophysiologic insomnia 123
Psychophysiological disorder 12, 114
Psychosexual
  disorders 134
  stage theory 20
Psychosis 12
Psychosocial treatments 58, 66
Psychotherapy 100, 105, 187
Psychotic
  disorders 52, 71, 74
  emergencies 166

R

Radio psychiatry 204
Rapid eye movement sleep 122
Recognizing hyperventilation syndrome 89
Recreational
  therapist 14
  therapy 198
Refusal of food 165
Regression 243
Relaxation
  techniques 234
  training 181
Repression 243
Reproductive system 226
Residual schizophrenia 55
Resolution of crisis 239
Respiratory
  disorders 127
  system 225
Restless leg syndrome 125
Rumination syndrome 115

S

Schizoaffective disorder 73
Schizoid personality disorder 132
Schizophrenia 5, 52, 53
Schizotypal personality disorder 132
Seasonal affective disorder 199
Second generation antipsychotics 173
Selection serotonin reuptake inhibitions 177

Senile dementia 68
Sensory system 36
Sequeeze technique 139
Serotonin hypothesis 54
Severe depression 166
Severity of psychosocial stressors 11
Sexual
  arousal disorder 136
  aspects of ageing 228
  aversion disorder 136
  behavior in elderly 229
  desire disorders 136
  dysfunction 136, 137
  pain disorder 136, 137
  response cycle 134
Shared psychotic disorder 74
Simple motor tics 154
Sleep
  apnea syndrome 124
  bruxism 126
  deprivation 128
  disorders 121, 126
  enuresis 126
  maintenance disturbance 127
  paralysis 126
  pattern disturbance 122
  starts 125
  talking 126
  terrors 125
  wake transition disorders 125
Social skills training 59
Somatization disorder 119
Somatoform disorders 86
Stages of
  dementia 70
  sleep 121
Stereotactic
  limbic leucotomy 84
  sub-caudate leucotomy 84
Stop start technique 139
Strategies of coping with stress 233
Stress 54
Structured interactions 189
Substance
  abuse 10
  dependence 215
  induced
    mood disorders 62
    psychotic disorder 74
  Act 171
Subtypes of schizophrenia 55
Suicide 162
Systematic desensitization 181

T

Tardive dyskinesia 175
Therapeutic
  activities 195
  communication 39
    techniques 43
  communities 133, 191
  graded exposure 183
  impasses 48
Thought disorder 57
Thyroid disease 68
Tic disorder 154
Transcutaneous electrical nerve stimulation 124
Transient ischemic attack 67
Treatment of
  acute polymorphic psychotic disorder with symptoms of schizophrenia 72
  alcohol dependence 100
  bipolar
    depression 65
    disorder 62
Tricyclic antidepressant 177
Tuberous sclerosis 144

Types of
  antidepressant 177
  anxiety 77
  ASDS 148
  aversion therapy 183
  crisis 238
  intervention 240
  mood disorders 60
  occupational therapy 195
  personality disorders 129
  psychotherapy 179

U

Urinary system 226

V

Vacuum pump 138
Vaginismus 136, 137
Viral infection 54
Vitamin deficiency 68

W

Warning signs of binge eating disorder 116
Wernicke-Korsakoff syndrome 68